Life beyond 1

Contents

I love you Nikki and Joshua Lee. Thanks for all of your support.

Life beyond the Scale
Introduction

It has no emotions, but it can control yours. It has no voice, but it can control how you speak to yourself. It has no eyes but can make you feel like it's looking inside your soul. It's always available to give you some attention, but it should rarely be paid attention to. You can stand on it with all your might, but it will often make you feel really weak. Do you know what I'm referring to? I'm talking about the dreaded scale!

It's incredible how this small device can have so much control over us. Depending on what the three digits are they can make a grown person cry! Have you ever struggled with the scale? Do you find yourself constantly drawn to it? Do you see yourself scared to get on it? Do you feel like you always need to know how much you weigh? Are you a SCALE-O-HOLIC, as one of my friends, described herself? If that's you, then it's time to go BEYOND THE SCALE!

For me, the scale has brought about a lot of stress. In fact, in 2016 I had two scales in my bedroom. My wife never used either of them. They were both for me. I know, I know, that sounds crazy, right? Well, it was. I had become so paranoid about where my weight was, and I wanted to be sure I had an accurate reading. I was measuring my success in the wrong way, as so many people often do. That's because as a society we've been conditioned to focus solely on the scale.

Watch television shows that deal with weight loss, and you will see that it's all about the scale. From the time we are born, we are put on the scale. While our childhood eventually comes to an end, our connection with the scale doesn't. It's time for us to lay aside the SCALE. It's time to start living beyond the SCALE.

I've heard a lot of people talk about their relationship with their scale. Some people I think spend more time on their scale than they do in the gym. I've heard things like…

"I weigh myself four times a day…"

"I weigh myself twice a week…"

I've even heard people use profanity when talking about the scale. WOW. Don't do that. A small little device can really do a number on our psyche. What about you? Are you ready to go beyond the SCALE? Let's go!

What I hope to accomplish with this book is to help you to break the vicious cycle of measuring your self-worth and accomplishments based upon what a stupid scale says to you. You are not a three-digit number. Don't let a number define who you are. It's not about the scale. While many people are seeking validation from the scale, what we need to be more concerned about is really living, and finding self-worth in the fact that we are made in the image of God.

So let's make an agreement. Don't get on the scale again until you have finished this book and the journal at the end (don't skip ahead and look either). Breathe now, please. I promise it will be okay if you don't weigh yourself for a few days. Ok, it will be more than a few days. More like a month or so. It will not take too long to read this. However, the journal at the end is where you may have the biggest challenge. But it will be worth it. As my friend Matt Bassford once said, "Some things are worth struggling through." I believe that when you are finished with this book, you will see it's not about the scale. You will have changed your mindset, which will allow you to lay aside the scale. There are some critical thoughts that I believe will help you to accomplish this.

1. We need to know why we should lay aside the scale.
2. We need to understand what it is that keeps us shackled to the scale.
3. What it will require for us to go beyond the scale.

Are you ready? Again, don't get on the scale until after you have finished this book. In fact, go ahead and throw away your scale or scales. If that last sentence gave you pause and produced fear in your heart, then you really need to lay aside the scale. Now you may be thinking, "Why should I listen to you?" That's a great question. I have had my struggles with my weight in the past. I am not a doctor. I am not a nutritionist. I did major in Kinesiology at the University of Illinois, and I am a certified health and wellness coach. You should always consult with a physician before beginning anything. Maybe, more importantly, is this: I have life experience. I know about the struggles of body image, overeating, and I know from experience how to lay aside the scale once and for all. I believe I have a talent of being able to motivate others. Hopefully, you will feel motivated to do more after reading this and to live life, beyond the scale. This book really began in 2016 when I started my physical transformation. Many of the ideas I will share with you were presented in two speeches I gave in March and April of 2017, at a fitness camp in Golden Colorado. I'm thankful for those opportunities I had during that time. I'm hoping this book will be able to help you and others. There will be some tips about what it takes to make a physical transformation. There is also a spiritual component in this book. As a Christian, I am proud of my faith. I think this element is often neglected when dealing with physical issues. So allow me to share my story with you as we prepare to live life beyond the scale.

Chapter One: A Love Affair with Exercise

"Ready, Set, Go..."

I've always had a love affair with exercise. I grew up in Urbana, Illinois, home of the Fighting Illini. I didn't have much stuff growing up. My dad was not around. You will learn more about him in a little bit. While me, my mom, and my sister didn't have much, I did have exercise. I had the outdoors. I had the playgrounds, the streets to run on, and weights to lift. I can remember as a young boy racing my friends on Busey Street in my Payless Shoes. Those shoes were cheap, but they were what we could afford during that time. I lost most of those races. But that didn't stop me. I have always loved to run. I may not have been the fastest, but that was okay. I didn't let my lack of athletic skills hold me back. I'm thankful my mother allowed me to be involved in sports. I can still recall the excitement, nerves, and thrills of participating in the presidential fitness test in grade school. I went to Yankee Ridge elementary school. I remember when I was in the fourth grade and introduced to this contest. It was great. It may have been the 600-yard dash that got me interested in running. Thinking back to that time, I can still feel the nervousness and anxiety I had right before the race began. That would carry over into every racing event I would do later. I received the presidential badge that year. But something happened in the fifth grade. I didn't hit the marks to receive another badge. Not getting another badge devastated me. Maybe that was preparing me for future disappointments in the sports arena. I tried to play football in middle school. That was a disaster. I had problems putting on the pads the proper way. I remember one game where I got hit in the throat. That was my sign that it was time to go. I would still be involved in football in the future, just in a different way. In high school, I was in the marching band. That would be the closest I would get back on the football field. I also played basketball in middle school, or at least I tried to. I think I averaged 0.8 points per game (that's not a typo) when I was in the eighth grade. That was an amazing year for us as a team. We went to state. We ended up getting fourth place. I cheered my team on from the bench since I rarely played. One of the coolest things I still remember about that year was the motto we had as a team. We had socks and towels made that said, "Get up." That phrase has stuck with me to this day. If you're friends with me on social media, you will often see me use this phrase. We all need a "Get up" type of mentality if we're going to be successful in accomplishing our goals. Somehow I made the freshmen and sophomore basketball teams. I can still remember how nervous I was when the coach would put up the list of the roster near the locker room at the school. There was a great sense of pride seeing my name on the roster, even if I didn't play that much. I ended up quitting the basketball team because I was wasting time sitting on the bench. One of the more memorable moments during my sophomore year playing basketball happened off the court. As I grew more frustrated with not being able to play, my mother decided to write the coach a letter. I was super embarrassed that she wrote the letter. But as I think about it, I'm impressed by how my mother supported me. When I look back at that moment, I realize that I wasn't that good when it came to basketball. There was a reason why I was on the bench. So I decided that homework would be more exciting instead of sitting on the bench. I traded in my basketball shoes for some running shoes. My junior year somehow I was persuaded to join the cross-country team. To this day, I still don't know how I was convinced into running cross-country. But I'm so happy that I did. It opened up another world for me. My fastest time for three miles was 18:06 during high school. That was good for me although there were other guys running sub 15 minutes in the three-mile race. I got to experience and appreciate what people call the runners high. I couldn't get enough of it. I remember the day after each race how I would pick up the daily newspaper to see if my name and time made it in the high school sports section. I was so thrilled when it was. I would cut out those clippings and keep them in a photo album. I still have them to do this day./

In high school, I was also introduced to weightlifting. At school, we had those old machines. I was weak, but I loved lifting. During that time someone bought me my first bench press. It was like a whole new world was unlocked in my mind. I'm not exaggerating when I say that I love to exercise. Some view exercise as some horrific burden. You will hear a lot of people say, "I got my workout done." What? What they should be saying is, "I was able to crush another workout today." People often fail when it comes to their fitness goals because of their mindset. We will work on that later on in the book. In high school, I continued to experiment with weightlifting. I wasn't doing anything super serious. Looking back at these early years is fun for me to do. If I could do it all over again, I probably would have given soccer a try. I would have worked harder and learned as much as I could about the sports I participated in. I am thankful however that I was able to do so much. Somehow the Lord provided the means for our family to have money for me to be involved in so many activities. We didn't have much money. The biggest reason why was because my father was absent from the home.

Chapter Two: Live and Learn or Learn and Live

I wish I could say that I was able to enjoy my love of exercise and fitness with my father. I wish I could say that my dad and I would play catch in the backyard after I came home from school. But I can't. Growing up my parents (at least when I was around) never owned a house. My dad and I never had those father and son moments that are often depicted in movies. That's because he wasn't around that much in my life.

While I have his eyes, I rarely was able to look into his. While I have his laugh, I rarely heard his laughter. While I have his last name, I did not really know the man behind the name. He was the man I knew and did not know. It has been seven years since my father died. I think writing about my father has become therapy for me. Talking to my mother about my father, I learned that he was a good man. My mom and dad were high school sweethearts (that's so cool). He was a hard worker. Looking at some old photos of him, he was definitely in shape. I learned that my dad came from a tough background. His mom had children from multiple men. He witnessed a lot of things that children should not see.

I don't recall my first memories with my father because he was not around much growing up. Looking back at all of the sporting events that I participated in, I don't recall my father ever being in the stands or on the sideline for any of them. My mother was always present for games. She was that mom who would always hug all of my teammates. As a young kid that was so embarrassing. It's super funny now. I don't believe my father ever attended any of my band recitals. The few memories that I have of him growing up are not the best. The first seven years of my mom and dad's marriage was great. He provided for his family well. He worked hard. I don't know when a change began for the worse in his life, but it was connected to him becoming a part of a bowling team. It's weird that it was related to some kind of sport. In the process of time, my dad began to do a lot of social drinking. That's what a lot of people do when they go to the bowling alley. They eat pizza, nachos, or chickens wings and throw back a couple of beers. Social drinking for my father turned into something much worse. He would become an alcoholic. It's interesting thinking about the memories I do have of my dad. I remember how he would cry more but only when he was drunk. His drinking escalated and would bring sorrow to our family. Obviously, since he was drinking that meant that he was out late at night. A lot of bad things happen after midnight. In time, he would cheat on my mother. He would also become physically and verbally abusive to my mother. I can still recall times where we had to stay at a woman's shelter for our safety. I can remember when we had to literally run away from our apartment in fear of what my father might do. I guess all of the running I did came in handy. Maybe the most vivid memory I have was on one particular night. I don't recall the month or the day. It was evening time. My parents were arguing. Arguing about what I have no idea. We were living on East Michigan Street in Urbana on the second floor of an apartment complex. My dad was drunk. He put his hands on my mother. In the process of time, he would pin her to the couch. I don't know if I was in my bedroom or not. Somehow I found myself in the living room where all of this was happening. Being young there was no way I was going to be able to pull my dad off my mother. So I did something else. I ran to the kitchen and grabbed a knife. It was a butter knife, but it was a knife nonetheless. I ran back into the living room and screamed as loud as I could. My scream startled my dad to the point where my mom was able to free herself from the couch. I honestly don't remember what happened after that. I know the people that lived below us called the police. I know that my mother was safe. I learned from my mother and sisters that after this incidence was when I began to sleepwalk. Strangely enough, I can still remember some of those nights when I slept walked. I can remember peeing on myself because I didn't pull my pants down when I went to the restroom. I can remember walking down the stairs at my grandparent's house, and thankfully they grabbed me before I walked out the door. I don't know how long I was in this sleepwalking stage. It may have been a year or so.

Oh yeah, I remember something else. I remember how bad of a temper I had when I was young. I think a lot of my anger issues stemmed from my father and maybe from that traumatic event that I witnessed. I should have received some type of counseling, but I never did. When I got angry as a child, I would often cry. But crying would only make matters worse. I would be mad about a variety of things. As a result, I received a lot of whoopings from my grandmother and my mom. I'm glad that I did.

Since my father was not around, it meant that my mom had to play the role of both mom and dad. She did an excellent job. It wasn't fair to her how more challenging her life became, but she handled it very well. As I mentioned earlier, we didn't have much. In fact, we had little. Not because my mother didn't work hard. It's because of my mother that I have a strong work ethic. She held a variety of jobs. She had office jobs and a range of home-based selling jobs. For a long period, she cleaned houses. My sister and I would often go along with her to help. I know how to clean toilets, windows, and a variety of other things because of those moments. During the summer we worked with mom cleaning many apartments. We called this "Turnover." When the college students moved out of apartments, we would go in and clean them before the new students moved in. I'm so impressed with my mother. I don't know how she got those contracts to do that, but she did. She hustled. My sister and I helped my mom clean those apartments. This meant no summer camps for us. I never attended any kind of summer camp until I became a counselor for a couple of years in my thirties. Those apartments were nasty and challenging to clean. It took forever for us to clean them. I believe my mom was working a full-time job. After getting off from that job, we would then tackle those apartments. We would clean until midnight or later on some nights. My mom was exhausted. So much so that in the process of time she would begin to have back issues. All of the physical labor eventually put her out of commission. She was on bed rest for many months. We were forced to begin using public aid. Random people assisted us by providing us with food at times. I still remember when we lived on East Michigan how one day there was this large food basket sitting at our apartment door. It was a reminder of how God always provides. Looking back I can laugh at the public aid cheese we would eat. That cheese was so thick. It would take forever for it to melt. But when it did, we chowed down on it. It made for some tasty grilled cheese sandwiches. I still love grilled cheeses (with honey on top). As I type this, I'm always amazed how we were able to survive. Even though dad was out of the picture, we still made it. My mother's parents who I called Granny and Papa provided a lot for us. They helped raise me. I also got a lot of whoopings from them. Yet I would learn a great deal about the Lord from them.

In the process of time, my father would come back into my life. Initially, I was not happy about it. My mother never got a divorce, although she had every scriptural right to. I was bitter about this for a long time. When I was told that mom and dad were getting back together, I was angry. I let my mother know how angry I was. When I had the opportunity to speak to my father, I also informed him how upset I was. During my junior year, while I was studying at the University of Illinois, I sat down with my father at a local Perkins restaurant. I didn't use any profane words, but I did let him have it. It was clear how I felt about him. I didn't trust him. He wasn't there for me when I needed him to be. He wasn't the one who took care of mom when she needed it. He wasn't the one who bought me my basketball shoes when I needed them. He wasn't the one cheering me on from the sidelines when I needed it. He wasn't there to teach me how to shave or put on a tie. He wasn't around to talk to me about girls and sex. He wasn't there to warn me about the dangers of pornography. He wasn't there. So, it was hard for me when suddenly he was there. What were we supposed to do? It wasn't like things were suddenly going to get back to normal. There was no normal. There had only been fear, chaos, and destruction when he was around. I was my own man now. I graduated from high school and would soon graduate from college. I didn't want mom and dad to get back together. But they did. Things seemed to work out well for some time. It was weird having another man around. I kind of filled that role. Eventually, my father and I would begin to spend more time together. Sunday dinners after morning worship were always a big deal for us. We would often go to my grandparent's house. We ate huge meals. I would call them naptime meals. That's because after you ate them, you would instantly want to take a nap. I can still smell the sweet potatoes with melted marshmallows and brown sugar, the baked turkey legs that looked like they came from some kind of dinosaur. I can taste the thick cornbread that I would pour honey over (I guess I really liked honey). I still see and taste the graham cracker cake my granny would make. It was like diabetes on a plate. The cake was filled with a ton of sugar. My grandfather absolutely loved them, and so did everyone else. If we weren't eating graham cracker cake, we were crushing huge oatmeal cookies. My granny could cook. All of the women in our family could and still can cook. My immediate family would begin to create some of our own memories. We were a complete family, although with problems. One thing that brought us together was food. However, our eating habits were not the best. I think many of us turned to food for comfort. We didn't know about the consequences of how we were feeding our bodies. Despite all of this it was a good time.

My father was not around during my early years, but I'm thankful he was available to see me graduate college. He was around to help me as I moved to Rockford, Illinois, for my first job out of college. I'm thankful that he was around long enough so we could make amends. There was one Sunday in particular that continues to stick with me. I was preaching at a small congregation in Urbana (more about my preaching later). I was talking about forgiveness. As I was teaching my mind went back to that conversation I had with my father at the Perkins restaurant. I thought about the way I had spoken to him that day. I thought about if I was genuinely honoring him as the scriptures teach, Ephesians 6:1-4. I thought about if I had truly forgiven him. He had tried to make amends. He was living differently. I needed to talk to him about this and make sure I was handling this situation correctly. We talked, and he told me that I had already discussed this with him. I genuinely don't remember that I had. But I guess I did. Mom and dad would stay together. They certainly had their ups and downs. Dad was back in the picture. He was around. Dad was there for me when I got married. He was there for me and my wife Nikki when we got our first house. Dad helped fix and put things together. He was there for us when we moved to Columbia Missouri. We had some fun times together. We tried to make the best of our situation. Having a son now, I should have had given more mercy and grace to my father. He was a flawed man like all of us are. He had his problems that stemmed from his childhood. He had a lot of issues that should have been resolved years earlier that weren't. I love my dad. My father had to fight alcoholism. He had to fight overcoming his temper that sometimes landed him in jail. In the process of time, he would have to fight cancer. My father's life would end as a result of throat cancer. It was tough seeing him go through all that he did. It was terrible seeing him lose so much weight and not being able to enjoy the foods that he loved so much. However, looking back I think getting cancer was the wake-up call that my father needed. My father needed to get right with the Lord. Facing death will do that to a person. My father died at the age of 59. He died way too young. I'm thankful that he was able to see his grandson. My son Joshua had very little time with him. I can see my dad in Joshua. My son has a loud voice like my dad. His laughter is distinct like my dad. I wish I could have been by my dad's side when he died. My sister and mother were. I learned a lot from my father.

- *I learned how fathers need to be in the picture.* Fathers have significant responsibilities, Ephesians 6:1-4. If you're reading this and are a father take some time and look back at some old photo albums. Are you in the pictures? Pictures are powerful. I love photo albums. When I finally got mine organized and began really looking at them carefully, I noticed how I only had a few pictures with my dad. As men, we need to be in the picture. We need to be around. We need to spend time with our children. Our children need to know that we will be there for them. Our wives need to know that we will keep them safe and provide for them. We can live and learn the hard way, or we can learn and live. Let's listen to God's word and fulfill our mission as men.

- *I learned how important health and nutrition really is.* My father didn't take care of his body. Like so many others, he got busy with work. For a while, he had a great job at Kraft. But with work, smoking cigarettes, drinking alcohol, poor eating habits, and lack of exercise, his body deteriorated faster than it should have. It was in no condition to fight cancer. I've learned that as a father I need to take care of my body. Our society talks about "Dad bods…" This is the idea of fathers who are out of shape. Society puts a lot of pressure on how people are supposed to look. Here's what I know. While dads don't need to look like a model or a professional athlete, we do need to take care of ourselves. It's hard to provide when we don't have our health. Who cares if you have a six-pack or not. We need to be more concerned about our blood pressure, cholesterol, and A1C levels. We need to take care of our bodies. We can live and learn the hard way or learn and live.

- *I learned that I don't want to have big regrets at the end of life.* I think all of us are going to have regrets. We get to decide how big those regrets are going to be. As I'm writing this, I am 40 years old. I have some regrets when I look back at the last 20 years of my life. One of the reasons why I'm writing this book is because I don't want to look back 20 years from now and say, "Why didn't I write that book? Who cares what people may have thought about it. Who cares if it only might have sold a few copies. I would have proven to myself that I could do it." I'm doing something right now, so I can avoid having that regret. My father had a lot of regrets as his time on this side of life came to an end. Regrets will be a part of life. But we get to decide how big those regrets may be. I get to choose how I'm going to treat my family. I get to decide how I'm going to take care of my body. While many things in life are out of our control, there are lots of things I can do avoid further regret. We get to decide how we want to learn this. We can live and learn the hard way, or we can learn and live. We can learn from others about what to do and what not to do. We can learn from the Holy Scriptures (read the book of Proverbs) and avoid a lot of future regrets.

I'm thankful for my father. I love my father. I have many of his traits and qualities. I look forward to seeing him in heaven.

Chapter Three: A Cup of Coffee That Changed My Life

"What do you want to do?"

When I graduated from high school in 1996, I enrolled at the University of Illinois. My love for fitness continued. I majored in Kinesiology. It was during this time when I really began to get serious about lifting weights and exercise in general. I would still have to learn the hard way. I had heard a lot about how much weight freshmen often gain. At the end of the first year, I became another statistic. There were a variety of bad decisions that I made my freshmen year. My family didn't have much money as I have already shared. Thankfully, my tuition was almost all covered by scholarships. The University of Illinois was in my hometown of Urbana. I should have lived at home while studying. But I didn't. I had to be grown and independent (and foolish). I decided to live in a dorm freshmen year. I stayed at Bromley Hall. It was a great dorm. The only problem was it was expensive. It was so expensive that I could only afford one meal per day in the cafeteria. Yep, that's right. I could have stayed at another dorm where I could have had three full meals a day covered. But I wanted this dorm. I got what I wanted but lost what I had (extra money). So, when it came time to eat, I ate. My roommate and I would eat a lot. In the cafeteria, there was this fruit juice that was available. We called it "fruity fruit juice." It was full of sugar, just the way I liked it. There were some glasses for us to use. So I would fill about six of those glasses up and drink all of them. My eating wasn't the best that year. But when you're young, you can often get away with eating bad foods. We would have pizza late at night or sometimes Burger King. One of the guys who stayed on my floor in the door was constantly eating Burger King Whoppers. I couldn't believe how many he ate. He ate whoopers and chewed tobacco. Clearly, he wasn't doing much schoolwork because he had to drop out at the end of the first semester. I don't think it was until my junior year until I really got serious about eating right. I had some weight to lose and thankfully I did. I was taking a swimming class that fall semester. It was early in the morning. I would bike to get to where the pool was, and then often swim for 45 minutes or so. I was burning a lot of calories. That gave me a lot of momentum to get back into shape and to keep the weight off. I had a great time during college. I continued with my running. I have great memories of going on late night runs on campus on the weekends. Back then I still had my cassette recorder with the big earphones compared to now. I listened to a lot of dance music. I wanted fast music to help keep me moving.

It was during college when I began working at a health club. This is probably a big reason why I have loved to go to a gym to workout. I began working at a Gold's Gym. I also did some part-time work at the school's workout facility. After I graduated, I became an assistant manager at the gym. That was a big deal for me. I laugh when I think about some of the things I did there. I would open up the gym around 5 or 5:30 a.m. I never had a problem getting there on time. I would get there early to ensure everything was set up. I would typically bring some leftovers and heat it up there. The only problem was the gym would smell like whatever food it was that I was eating. This wasn't good, especially if it was Chinese Food. I loved Chinese Food, but it wasn't always the healthiest. I feel bad how so many of the members who came to get an early morning workout were greeted with this smell of bad food. Oops! During this time I really focused on getting stronger. It worked. I was bench-pressing 325 pounds weighing around 175 pounds. That was really good for me. What wasn't good for me was how much caffeine I began to consume. There was an energy drink called "Razor" that we sold at the gym. I loved it. It was a dollar, and it got me moving. Eventually, that drink disappeared from the market. It didn't matter. I used other stimulants like Ripped Fuel. I couldn't believe how much I would sweat using that product. I also found another energy drink called "Speed Stack." I was using these all of the time. As I reflect upon the last 20 years, I recognize that I have consumed way too much caffeine. I went from Razors to Speed Stacks, to Rip Fuel, to Five-hour energy, and to coffee. Caffeine is good, but there's a limit. One can go too far with stimulants, and I think I did. I never used steroids. I couldn't afford them, and I was too afraid to. I know there were some at the gym who were on steroids. After a while, I was able to point them out. During this time, I also became a certified Spinning Instructor and did some personal training along the way.

Working at the health club caused me to go a little overboard. I would teach spin classes with my shirt off. Before there were selfies, I was doing selfies. It's safe to say that I was obsessed when it came to exercise and fitness. How I looked is what would consume me. I can remember asking my mom and sister to take photos of me while I flexed. I know, I know, it was over the top. I'm happy I had the opportunity to be able to work at a health club. I learned so much. I learned…

- ***One must put time and energy to stay in shape.*** Those who are consistent will succeed. Those who aren't will not. There was one man at the gym who I still admire to this day. He lost 100 pounds in a year. It was so inspirational to see him come in day after day and get on a Stairmaster. I remember talking to a young woman at the gym and asking her how she always found a way to get her workout in. She responded by saying, "You just have to do it. You have to find a way to get it done." That's the mindset that we're after. That's the mindset we must have if we are going to go beyond the scale.

- ***When you work hard, people will notice.*** I was asked to be a part of a fitness book called "Mind and Muscle: Psych Up, Build Up." Being able to be a part of a fitness book was such a big deal for me. I couldn't believe it. Now before you think I was on the cover or anything like that, I wasn't. I had two pictures in the book where I was working out. That gave me a massive boost in confidence. It helped me to maintain the drive, focus, and consistency to stay in great shape and to work towards hitting a goal.

Working at Gold's Gym was not the only exposure I had to fitness. My junior year in college I was able to take part in a Summer Research Opportunities Program. I helped one of my professors who was testing walking pedometers. We would take people out on the quad and measure their steps. I had no idea how valuable those devices would become. I wish I had the vision to see the opportunities that were potentially available for me during that time. But I wasn't really thinking about the big picture. I was focused on getting my lifts in and staying lean. I had a variety of other jobs during college, like working at Walgreens. But the majority of what I did was still connected to fitness. It's incredible seeing how connected I've been to fitness as I look back. While I majored in Kinesiology, I didn't know what I wanted to do. For a while, I thought I would become an athletic trainer where I would work with a collegiate or professional team. I was accepted into the sports training program and had an opportunity to work with the women's swim team for a while. But after spending a short time as a trainer, I decided to opt out of the program. I didn't want to do it. But I did want to stay connected to fitness. I just didn't know exactly what. But there would be a day while I was working at Gold's Gym that would change my trajectory. I got into a conversation with one of the guys at the gym that I knew. One day he asked me a question. He asked me what it was that I wanted to do after I graduated. My response was, "I have no idea." I really couldn't go too much further with the position I had at the gym. I was helping others reach their fitness goals, but at the same time, I was feeling restless. Okay, let me change that. I was feeling broke! I wanted and needed more money. And in all seriousness, I knew that there was more out in the world for me to do.

I feel terrible that I can't remember the name of the man who I talked to. He was such a nice guy. He took time out of his schedule to have some coffee with me. He shared with me what he did. He was a pharmaceutical sales rep. He worked for Merck, which was one of the biggest companies at the time. Having a cup of coffee with him would put me on a new course in my life. I don't know what he saw in me, or why he took the time to help me, but I'm thankful he did. From that conversation, I took the plunge to see if I could get a job in sales. I never thought I would be a drug dealer! Ok, that's a stretch. But I guess you can say that I desired to be a promoter of life-saving products.

My prayer was answered after receiving an offer from Pfizer Inc. Man, talk about a big move up from working at a local health club to now selling billion-dollar products. Looking back at this transition, I can see that I kept a connection with health and fitness. While I was no longer going to be training people how to lift dumbbells, I would be training and teaching physicians about life-saving products. My love affair with fitness and health continued.

Chapter Four: A Medicine Many Don't Want

"You have two options: You can continue to take your pills, or you can exercise and eat healthily and eliminate all of your pills. Which one do you want?"

This was a question a physician shared with me during a lunch one day in Rockford Illinois. He was an endocrinologist. I brought him in to talk to some of my physicians. He shared how he would often pose this question to his patients. Sadly, the reply from so many of his patients was that they would rather take pills, instead of adopting a healthy approach with diet and exercise.

Isn't that weird? Isn't that sad? The one thing people need, want, and can have is HEALTH. Yet, so many times we decide not to do the very things we need to do. Too many want to take the easy way out, instead of working hard. I don't know if I'm the only one who has made this correlation, but I think in America we have become much like what's seen in the movie WALL-E. Have you seen that movie? It's funny. And yet, it's a little scary. Everyone in the film was fat and lazy. They didn't exercise. They ate and ate and ate. They didn't even walk. They had to relearn how to walk because they were so dormant. When I watched that movie, I couldn't help but think, "This is what's happening in America!"

As we talk about living life beyond the scale, we need to recognize the power of exercise. So many people want some quick diet plan that will shed the weight without exercise. There are plenty of options available if you really want to lose weight fast. But that's all you will really do. You will lose the weight really fast, but you will eventually find the weight again. We don't want to lose the weight, but rather as my sister told me, "We want to release the weight" once and for all. That will mean that we will have to go beyond the SCALE. We're not looking for quick fixes, but sustainable things we can do for life. We will need to eat well and exercise. That's because it's not just about the number on the scale. It's about LIFE. It's about genuinely LIVING. Therefore, exercise is critical.

I've heard many people say, "EXERCISE is medicine." That's so true. Exercise is powerful. It can change your mood. It's a great way to get the juices flowing for thoughts and creativity. It makes you feel and look better. Someone once said, "Exercise is a medicine with great side effects." Do you believe this to be true? I do. I learned this early on in life. Through exercise,

I could release a lot of my anger. It changed my mood. It continues to do the same for me now. Walking into doctor offices and seeing physicians overweight and so many patients suffering had a profound impact on me. Many of the illnesses people suffered from could have been avoided if the patients would have chosen a better lifestyle. While it's easy to look at others and tell them what they need to do, it can be hard to gaze in the mirror and see what we need to do. Now, I know it's easy to say all of this, but it is often harder to actually do.

I will be the first to admit, that at times I have been a hypocrite. When I was with Pfizer, selling cholesterol drugs, blood pressure drugs, and diabetes products, I allowed my health to decline. I eventually had to take one of my own medicines. Grief. What a hypocrite right? It can happen so quickly. I didn't have the proper mindset during a lot of my time while in sales. I was so focused during my last few years in college and when I first started with Pfizer. But I allowed life to get in the way. All of those dinner programs and lack of discipline on my part began to show on my waistline. To make matters worse, I was still very connected to the scale. Eventually, I stopped trying to be diligent in my eating and exercise. I played the blame game. I began to use excuses, which took away my health. I lied to myself with excuses like...

1. "I'm driving so much, and I don't have time to exercise."
2. "I need to eat this food at these dinner parties."
3. "I've been in shape for so long, taking a little bit of time off and getting out of shape will not hurt me."
4. "I can work out extra, and I will be okay even though I'm eating terribly."

It's so easy to deceive ourselves. It's so easy to think we can get away from doing the fundamental things that need to be done. Being in shape takes work. The work is worth it. We just have to get our mindset in the right place to really believe this to be true.

We will need to view exercise as medicine. We need to embrace the power of it, and how it will positively affect our lives for the better. I would come to really understand the importance of my health a few years later when I moved from Rockford, Illinois, to Columbia, Missouri.

Chapter Five: "You Have HCM..."

"I'm invincible! I can't be touched."

That was the mindset I had in college and in my early twenties. As I mentioned earlier, I was benching 325 pounds and weighing 175 pounds. I had my six-pack! I was in great shape. I would meet my future wife Nikki in Syracuse New York in 2003. I was living in Rockford Illinois at the time. She was living in Fort Lauderdale Florida. We met at an event called "Campaign for Christ." We both traveled to do some work at a local congregation in Syracuse New York. We would door knock and hold Bible studies during the day. At night, we would gather for a sermon. It was during this time that I would sweep Nikki off of her feet. At least that's the story that I share when people ask how we met. The truth is I was a little slow in the sense that it took me a while to see that she was interested in me. Eventually, I asked her out one evening to go somewhere to get some dessert. It's funny looking at the connections and similarities we shared. One was with our names. Nikki's maiden name was Benjamin. What are the odds of that? That was enough reason for us to get married. Okay, not really, but it is pretty interesting. My minister at the time used to be Nikki's youth minister growing up. What are the odds of that? And now we were both in New York doing the work of the Lord. What could be better? That first night I asked her out we went to Friendly's Restaurant. One of the sisters was with us as well. My preacher and his family were there, but sitting in another booth. They kept giving me a thumbs up sign as they saw me sitting and talking with Nikki. Nikki and I would talk a lot that week. I learned some weird things about her. She was really into dental floss. I still laugh when I think our conversations about dental floss. One evening while I was driving her home we got on the conversation about marriage. During that conversation, I mentioned to her that she might be sitting next to her future husband. Looking back, that was a pretty bold statement. I'm surprised she didn't jump out of the car. When it came time for me to leave, we exchanged information. I tell people that she gave me all of her information (phone number, pager number, social security number, address, etc.). She always gets upset when I mention that. She didn't give me all of her information, but a lot of it. When I drove back to Rockford Illinois with my preacher and his family, his son asked me a question. He asked me, "Is Nikki your girlfriend?" I think I told him, no, but I wish she would be. All of this took place in August of 2003.

Nikki and I would talk quite a bit on the phone. We would talk for hours. That's all we could do since I was in Illinois and she was in Florida. During one of those conversations in the weeks after we met, we got on a discussion of pedicures and manicures. How we began to talk about pedicures and manicures, I have no idea. Eventually, I told her, "We need to go and get a pedicure and manicure together." I think she laughed and then said, "How are we going to do that?" I told her, "Well, obviously I would have to fly there to do it." That's what I did. Our first date was getting pedicures and manicures. I still remember when Nikki picked me up at the airport what she was wearing. She had on these white pants. She was beautiful and still is. Our first kiss was at the airport. I stayed a few days and then had to fly back for work. We would continue to talk on the phone. We also wrote letters to one another. I still remember a photo Nikki sent me. It was taken at her job. She was wearing a brown top and skirt and was beautiful. We met in August. I proposed in October. I flew to Florida to talk to her dad and to get his permission before I asked her to marry me. She knew it was coming because we had begun to do some ring shopping in Rockford when she arrived and visited (we stayed in separate places when visiting to eliminate the temptation of sexual immorality). I decided on two options concerning how I was going to propose to her. My first option was for us to play the board game life. Whenever we landed on family or marriage (I can't remember what exactly is on the board), I would propose. But I decided to go plan B. I would propose on the beach. The only problem was Nikki was not interested in going to the beach. She lived next to the beach her entire life, so going there was not really a big deal. Eventually, I persuaded her to take us there. By then it was getting dark. It was windy as well. I got on one knee, and through wind and sand in my eyes, I asked her to marry me. Of course, she said yes. We would get married the following year in Rockford Illinois. There were so many things that attracted me to Nikki. First, she was a Christian. I loved the fact that we met doing the work of God. Second, she loved to eat. Yes! Third, she loved to workout. When we met, she was running about four miles a day. Finally, she loved football. What else could a man ask for? Oh yeah, did I mention that she is beautiful? After we got married, we stayed in Rockford Illinois for another year. I was still with Pfizer and eventually got a job promotion to Columbia Missouri. Overall, life was good. We bought our first home in Illinois. We would buy another house when we moved to Columbia Missouri. We had a health scare on our honeymoon in Florida. The first day of our honeymoon, Nikki felt a lump in one of her breasts. We both began to worry. Thankfully, it turned out to be nothing. But a few years later, I would get a health scare. It would be something. It would be life-changing.

While living in Columbia, Missouri, I went in for a routine physical. The nurse practitioner asked if I wanted an EKG. I said, "Is it covered by my insurance?" She said, "Yes" and then I said, "Yes, let's do it." That's when things would change forever. The nurse practitioner said, "Your T-Wave is inverted." That's not good. That would be the beginning of a lot of doctor's appointments.

I would go on and have a series of visits with my local cardiologist, a cardiologist at Washington University in St. Louis, and finally, I saw another specialist at the Minneapolis Heart Institute in Minnesota. The diagnosis: HCM. HCM stands for Hypertrophic Cardiomyopathy. I know you're probably thinking, "What is that?" I didn't know what it was either when I first heard about it. The short story is I have abnormal thickening in a portion of my heart. People who have this genetic condition have excessive thickening, which is why the word hypertrophy is used. This thickening is found in the left ventricle. For more information about this condition check out this website (www.4hcm.org). My life was changing right before my eyes. It appeared that my love affair with exercise was about to vanish. I never thought I had a problem. I never really had any symptoms. Now, instead of being fired up to go to the gym, I was scared. Would I go into cardiac arrest? Would I drop dead on the treadmill? As I processed more of what was taking place, and having more conversations with my physician, I realized that I could still exercise. However, I would have to change what I typically did. Gone were the heavy lifting days. Gone were the competitive activities. At least that's what I was told and recommended. Needless to say, I was a little stubborn. After my diagnosis, I walked a ½ Marathon. My physician did not advise this, but I did it anyway. I was beating people walking. It was hard to walk the race instead of running it. I felt like I was being robbed of my LIFE. Having this condition was not fair. But looking back, I realize how blessed I really was and have been.

"You're T-Wave is inverted…"

"You have Hypertrophic Cardiomyopathy…"

"There's one word to describe your condition…UNPREDICTABLE…"

Isn't interesting how some statements really stick with you? I will never forget those words and the moments they were uttered. So, after being diagnosed with HCM, I had to make some long-term decisions. Many with HCM decide to get an ICD (Implantable Cardioverter Defibrillator). While it doesn't happen often, some with HCM will experience sudden cardiac arrest. After much prayer, fear, and consultation, I decided to get an ICD planted in my chest. Talk about a game changer. My chest would never look the same. Now I have a scar and a slight bulge on my right side of my chest. I experienced a lot of doubt and fear during that time. I was in a preacher-training program not making a lot of money. I knew I was going to have a massive hospital bill. I began to contemplate if I should get back into secular work. The hospital bill came back: $80,000. I had recently been severed from Pfizer Inc. Thankfully part of the severance package was keeping my health insurance for a while. I only ended up paying about $1,000 out of pocket. God is good not just some of the time, but all of the time.

I had my first ICD placed in 2010. I felt like Iron Man afterward (just without all of the power and money). I had to take about six weeks off from physical activity. When I was able to jog again, I remember the first time I went out to run, and I fell. Talk about bad luck. I instantly thought that I had ruined my new device. Fear crippled me for a long time. I had a hard time lifting dumbbells over ten pounds in the gym. I often thought to myself, "I'm never going to be able to get anywhere at this pace." I didn't even do push-ups for many years after receiving my device. Gone were my heavy reps on the bench press.

But in the process of time, I decided that I couldn't live in fear any longer. Note: For those who have an ICD and are reading this I created a motivational journal for you. It's called, "I CAN DO: A motivational journal for people with an ICD." I decided to change what ICD means to me. If you find yourself struggling to get back to exercise, you will have to do the same. This journal is available on Amazon and my website www.benjaminleeonline.com.

I followed protocol and got back into the grove of lifting. Yet in life, there will always be some kind of obstacle that you will have to overcome. To go beyond the scale, you must be prepared to fight when life tries to knock you down. I know by experience. I had finally begun to overcome the fear of having an ICD, only to have another fear arise. It happened in June of 2014. I was at the gym warming up on the treadmill. I was jogging at a slow pace, around 6 m.p.h. About five minutes into my jog I began to feel weird. Suddenly, all of my teeth started to throb. I began to sweat profusely. I immediately became exhausted. I've never had a heart attack, but if I were, this is what it would probably feel like. I got off the treadmill. I should have had someone call 911 for me, but I was stubborn. I sat there for minutes in shock. My ICD had not shocked me. The pain wasn't going away. Eventually, I drove (yes that was a bad idea) myself to an urgent care clinic. I told them I thought I may be having a heart attack (yep, that was dumb) and they said there wasn't much they could do for me. I called my wife to come to pick me up. We didn't immediately go to the E.R. In all honestly, I was thinking more about how much all of this was going to cost me. That's why I delayed going to the hospital. Instead, we went to one of those emergency care clinics. They are bigger than a regular urgent care but smaller than a hospital. Initially, my blood work came back normal. But a few hours later my troponin levels came back elevated. I was told that it appeared that I had a heart attack. How could this be? I'm too young to have a heart attack. In fact, that's what I would hear during the weeks following this event. It turned out that I didn't have a heart attack. Instead, I had a blood clot in my right coronary artery. Ouch. I was devastated. What did this mean? I had to start over again. I went to cardiac rehab and walked super slow on the treadmill. That was the easy part. The hard part was the mental battle I was facing again. But in the process of time, I would decide that I couldn't live in fear. I had to keep pressing forward. I was put on a blood thinner and continue to take it. But four years later thank the Lord I'm still here. But I again struggled with the scale. My mindset was still not in the place where it needed to be. Even though I could work out, I never felt like I could get back to the intensity I once had. I wasn't doing what I needed to do with my eating. I merely focused on exercise. I've discovered that my mindset at the time was in the wrong place. I had this limiting belief that I could eat terribly and as long as I worked out things would be okay. FALSE! That's a blind spot that a lot of people have. You can't outwork a bad diet. In the process of time, I would learn that.

Chapter Six: Please Pray That I Get Severed

"We thank you for your services with Pfizer, but we no longer need them."

Ok, I don't think it was said exactly like that when I got the call that I was being let go with Pfizer in January of 2009, but I think that statement is close. I mentioned earlier that I had gotten severed from Pfizer. After eight years with the number one company in Pharmaceutical Sales, I was being let go. YES. Thank you, GOD! That's not an exaggeration. Let me tell you why.

Remember that restless feeling I told you about while I was working at the gym? It came back. I don't know what you would call it. But I just had a feeling that it was time for me to go and to do something bigger. The pharmaceutical industry had evolved significantly from when I began in 2001. It was becoming increasingly more difficult to have contact with physicians. The money was great. In hindsight, I took for granted everything I had while I worked for Pfizer. They took good care of me. That job forced me to get out of my comfort zone. I learned so much about the world and how business works. But there was something bigger I needed to do. But what might that be? What could be more significant than working at a health club or with a billion-dollar pharmaceutical company? Wait for it...ARE YOU READY...Okay, here it is... PREACHING THE WORD OF GOD!

Some may be laughing right now! Some may be thinking, "You went into preaching? Why would you take that career path?" Let me explain how I got to this point. I've had a lot of preachers in my family. My grandfather was a preacher. I have an uncle who is still preaching. I never thought that I would be a preacher, but never say never.

As a young boy, I would preach from time to time (if you really want to call it preaching). I grew up in a real small church of about 10 people. Yep, told you it was a small church. We had one cup when it came time to partake of the Lord's Supper. We had no Bible classes. We would drive from Urbana Illinois to Indiana to worship with a few people there on Sundays. We believed that we had to use wine for the Lord's Supper and not grape juice. I remember making a radio commercial where I invited people to services and how I emphasized what we had for the Lord's Supper. Now, I believe we had a misunderstanding of some scriptures concerning the wine being used for the Lord's Supper and the one-cup. My definition of preaching at the time was gathering some verses from the concordance at the back of the Bible, and then reading them and then sitting down. BOOMS…drop the mic. The only thing that dropped was probably the morale of the people in the room after trying to figure out what exactly I was trying to say.

In Rockford, Illinois, I got a chance to really preach for the first time. My first sermon was called "One More Night With The Frogs." It was a great lesson! It was great because it wasn't mine. I stole it from another preacher. I confess my sin, <u>James 5:16</u>. I mean I took it word for word. I had a lot of drive time while I was in sales. I would spend a lot of my time listening to sermons (this was in the days of cassette tapes). Somehow I heard this lesson. The rest is history. However, I would learn my lesson about using someone else's material. It may come back to bite you. A few months after I preached that sermon, our congregation held a gospel meeting. A gospel meeting is when a visiting preacher comes in and teaches on a particular topic or topics for about a week. Can you guess who the visiting preacher was that year? Yep. It was the man who wrote the sermon I stole. I can't make this up. I attended each night of the meeting. I was scared each night I was going to be exposed as a fraud. I sat in the pew with fear and trembling. I prayed that he wouldn't preach that sermon. I never had the nerve to tell him I used his sermon. Thankfully, he never preached it. A few years ago my aunt sent me a copy of that sermon. I listened to it and couldn't believe what I was hearing. It was awful. I couldn't even finish listening to my own sermon. Thankfully, I've grown since that time. I've also grown when it comes to using someone else's material. I write my own sermons. If I use someone's idea, I will ask and give them credit.

Needless to say, I didn't have a lot of tools or confidence to think that I should preach. But something changed between Rockford and Columbia. I saw the great need for preachers. Let's face it, how many men are saying that they want to be a preacher? Exactly. Many brethren joke about how preachers only work five hours a week. If that was the case, then preaching would be the perfect job for guys to have. You could work five hours and then get to do whatever you wanted to the rest of the week. We know that is not the case. I felt the need to preach. I was growing tired with Pharmaceutical Sales. I didn't feel like I was making an impact on the world, as much as I could. I didn't hear a small still voice that was telling me to preach. I didn't have a vision or anything like that. I saw a need. I walked by faith.

The brethren in Columbia, Missouri, were so great to Nikki and me. For some strange reason, they gave me an opportunity also to preach after the local preacher moved. Again, I had no idea what I was doing. But an opportunity opened up. I was still in sales. But eventually, I began praying that God would open a door for me to preach full time. That door would be opened. It's interesting how God opens up doors. It's often not in the way that we think.

I would be let go by Pfizer so that I could go preach the gospel. I may have been the only person celebrating on that Friday morning after being told that I no longer had a job. When God opens doors, He will open them big. I believe in the Providence of God. I know that sometimes things happen by coincidence, but God is still working. Our God is alive. He always answers prayer. That's why we need to pray big. I did, my family did, and my church family did. I asked my congregation to pray that I get let go by Pfizer. You should have seen their faces when I made that request. But listen, we should be specific in our prayers. When you read 2 Corinthians 12:7-9, you see that the apostle Paul was very clear and direct in his prayers. We should follow his example. While God may have something else in mind, we need to be bold in our prayers. Too many Christians pray small. We don't serve a little God, but one who is big. Take some time to read Luke 11:1-13 and 18:1-8. Take a minute and really think about these questions.

- How does Jesus teach us how to pray?
- What kind of confidence should we have in our heavenly Father?

My prayer was answered. But how you may ask? I'm so glad you asked, let me tell you. While in Columbia Missouri, I learned about a local church in Beaumont, Texas. That congregation was the Dowlen Road Church of Christ (www.dowlenroad.com). They had a preacher trainer program, where they would bring in a young man and teach him how to preach. This is following the pattern of 2 Timothy 2:2, where older men teach the younger men. The congregation had been looking for a young man for about a year. Three previous men had already completed the program. Things were beginning to line up for me. I knew that my days with Pfizer were limited. It was time to go. Better to have a plan before I was officially let go. I needed an exit strategy. I was thinking about going to Arkansas to a Bible school, but my wife didn't want to move there.

So I inquired about the preaching program in Beaumont. I thought to myself, "Can anything good come out of Beaumont?" YES. A lot of good came out of Beaumont. Nikki and I flew down for a weekend to talk to the Shepherds of the congregation. The discussion went really well. I would get the offer to come to Beaumont. I took it. But I still needed to be let go from Pfizer. I guess I could have quit the company if for some reason I wasn't let go. But by being let go, I received a nice severance package. Nikki and I made two good salaries while in Missouri. For a while, we had little to no debt. But sadly, we were often unwise with the money we made. So getting the severance package was a good thing. When we moved to Beaumont, we moved paying off all our debts. We were also blessed that we were able to sell our home. This was in 2009, so the housing market was terrible. It was not a seller's market. We broke even. I didn't want to move to Texas and worry about a house in Missouri. God again answered our prayers.

As a couple, we were about to experience what I call our Abraham and Sarah moments. Are you familiar with the story of Abraham and Sarah? If you know the story of those two and the promises God gave to Abraham, then you will have a good understanding of what the Bible is all about.

A man named Abraham and his wife Sarah were told by God in Genesis 12:1-3, to go to a land that they had never been to. God promised Abraham (there are more than three promises)…

- That he would give him a land, Genesis 12:1.
- That he would make him a great nation, Genesis 12:2.
- That in him all families of the earth would be blessed, Genesis 12:3.

Nikki and I had our first Abraham and Sarah moment moving from Illinois to Missouri. I don't mean that the Lord audibly spoke to me. But instead, we believed that God was working in our lives and that this was the place He wanted us to be. This would be a move of faith like it was for Abraham and Sarah. We sold our house. I was making $88,000 a year with Pfizer, company car, excellent benefits, and moving to Beaumont with a salary of $25,000 waiting for me. Ouch. The congregation in Missouri also supported us financially some for our first year. While our finances were changing, it would be worth it. This was an opportunity I could not ignore. Remember what I mentioned earlier about regret? I didn't want to look back years later and say, "You should have tried that preacher training program."

We moved because life is about challenges. Too many people stay in the same place. Too many are afraid to FAIL. We can't be scared to fail. Life is about failing, learning, and trying again. Looking back at all of this I can see that this was just another learning process for me to get to this point of writing this book, going beyond the scale, and helping so many who struggle with poor health, etc.

I honestly didn't know if this preaching program would work. I was told that if I weren't a good fit, then I would be let go. That made me a little fearful. But the things that we fear the most rarely happen! Nikki and I survived. In fact, we did more than just survive. We thrived. We made the adjustment with the lower salary although it was difficult. We were humbled and were able to learn a lot. I never thought how far the move from Columbia Missouri to Beaumont, Texas, would take us.

The preaching program lasted for two years. It was tough but enjoyable. I had two great mentors. I love those men very much. During the training program, I learned how to write sermons, put together workbooks, how to present sermons, teach Bible class, and so much more. I learned the value of excellent leadership. Nikki and I developed lasting relationships with the brethren. The two years flew by. I was extremely sad thinking about the idea that I would have to leave and begin working at another congregation. In 2011, God worked in another significant way. All of the previous men who entered the training program left to go work with another group. That's how it's designed. But I was asked if I would be willing to stay full time and work with the congregation. Again, God did something that I never thought would happen. I had thought to myself during the program, "How cool would it be if I were able to stay at Dowlen Road and preach full time." My thoughts became a reality. VERY COOL! I was asked to stay as a full-time preacher. Of course, we accepted. Nikki and I were thrilled beyond measure. Some may think, "Wow, three preachers is a lot." We have examples like in Acts 13:1, where the church in Antioch of Syria had multiple teachers. There's much work to do a local congregation. Dowlen Road is a large congregation as well, so there was plenty to do. I was able to work at the Dowlen Road congregation from 2009–2018. I'm a blessed man. I experienced a lot during my time in Beaumont, Texas. During that time…

- I received two new ICD's (Implantable Cardioverter Defibrillator)
- Nikki and I experienced the joy of having our son named Joshua.

- I experienced the death of my father and grandparents, along with other family members. Nikki also suffered death among her families.
- I've was able to preach the gospel in South Africa, Zimbabwe, Botswana, Mexico, and in Missouri, Arkansas, Louisiana, New York, Florida, Mississippi, Indiana, Minnesota, Colorado, and Alabama.
- I've seen many men and women become new creatures in Christ by believing in Jesus Christ and being baptized for the forgiveness of sins, <u>Acts 2:38</u>; <u>Mark 16:16</u>.

I was able to experience so much. I'm thankful for all of the relationships I was able to experience and the influence that I've had upon others. It is truly humbling. As a preacher once said to me, "God is good, not just some of the time, but all of the time."

Chapter Seven: You Work Out and Still Have a Belly

"You workout and still have a belly."

That's what Nikki told me one day while I was ironing a shirt. I had gotten back home from the gym. I was feeling good about myself. I felt strong. That would quickly change. I showered and made my protein shake. I had put on some muscle (even though it was hidden under FAT). While ironing Nikki looked at me in my undershirt and said "You workout and still have a belly." I was taken aback for a few seconds. I chuckled a nervous laugh. Then I went into defense mode.

ME: "Oh, yeah but I'm gaining muscle."

NIKKI: "Yeah, but aren't you supposed to be in shape since you go to the gym so much?"

ME: "UMMMMM…yeah..."

So what happened? I believed a BIG LIE that many others believe. Many think that they can eat whatever they want and believe exercise will cover up for their loose lips and binge eating of food. So not true. Eventually, that kind of mindset will sink you. It does every single time.

I had bought into the lie. I worked out for the most part on a consistent basis. I would have days where I would miss one or two days. But my EATING wasn't right. There were some other lies I had believed. I thought taking supplements would make up for my poor eating habits. NOPE. WRONG. LIE. My mindset wasn't where it needed to be. And I was still connected to the scale. My success was measured on the scale. At the time I wasn't having much success with it either. That will often create a slippery slope. I would fall further into the abyss due to a lack of self-control. This became really evident to me in February of 2016. I would eat a two-pound donut. Yep, that's right. It's not a typo. I had been watching a lot of episodes of Man vs. Food. I told myself, "Self, you should try that." Austin Texas is only about five hours from Beaumont Texas. I heard about a donut shop called Round Rock Donuts. They had a two-pound donut. I had to try it. Okay, I didn't have to try it. Someone should have slapped me. I should have slapped myself. Eating this donut was an insane thing to do. But I would do it anyway. My family and our friends went on a little road trip. Normal people go on a road trip to visit the Statue of Liberty or Mount Rushmore. Others take a road trip to run some kind of marathon or something. Not me. I went on a trip to eat a big fat donut. I accomplished my mission, although it felt like death. I finished the donut in about 45 minutes. I think it was equivalent of eating a dozen donuts. The first half was actually enjoyable. The second half I had to walk around and literally force myself to finish. To make matters worse later on that day we all went out to lunch. I had pizza and then followed it up with some ice cream when we got to our rental home. WHOA. Can you say out of control? This began a downward spiral for me with my weight. I knew I was fat, but I didn't know just how fat. I had moments like these in the past. I remember dating a woman while in Rockford Illinois before I met Nikki. I was on this cycle of eating a ton of calories for two weeks and then cutting calories for two weeks. The goal was to gain muscle mass while keeping the fat off. The only problem was I wasn't following the eating regiment. Instead of sweet potatoes and oatmeal for carbohydrates, I was eating whole pizzas. My girlfriend once said to me, "You're getting fat." I shook it off. I thought I was in control. I wasn't. Now, years later I was doing it again. I just didn't want to admit it. I certainly didn't want to get on the scale either. You see, like so many other people I was afraid of the scale. Silly me, I had plenty of other indicators that were screaming at me and saying, "DUDE, WHAT ARE YOU DOING?"

Consider exhibit #1: CLOTHES

"Clothes Don't Lie." That's a saying I have with some of my friends. I have a brown suit. It had been in Illinois for a while at my mom's place. In 2016, my clothes kept getting tighter. I was getting fatter. I eventually forced myself to get on the scale. Oh boy…I weighed in at 239. WHAT! I had never weighed that much in my life. Feeling disappointed was an understatement. I was crushed. How could I let myself get so out of shape? I was outgrowing my suits. I decided to have my mom send me my brown suit. This was the brown suit that I had left in Illinois after a family visit. When I left it there, I was calling it my fat suit. I was sure that I could fit into this suit with no problem, and I didn't want to go and buy another suit. But I would be devastated after getting it. I couldn't get into it. When I tried it on, I couldn't even BUTTON IT UP. NNNNNOOOOOO…

I was experiencing as one of my friend's calls it "Dunlap's disease." This is when your belly has Dun Lapped over your belt. Yep, I was guilty.

Consider exhibit #2: COMMENTS

I guess I should have been more aware of my weight problem when a friend of mine yelled across the church parking and said, "Looks like you are getting wider."

A sister at church kept telling me how disappointed she was with me for allowing myself to get where I was. I had played the role of the hypocrite. I had been telling her a few years earlier about staying in shape. She was at risk for diabetes. Now it was her turn to help me.

Consider exhibit #3: NO CONFIDENCE

I had lost a lot of confidence in myself. I wasn't happy with my body. I didn't like how I looked or felt. All of these pieces of evidence were beginning to add up.

What a stinking failure. I felt like I had hit rock bottom. I had tried working with a nutritionist I believe back in 2015 who put me on a rigorous eating plan. I mean it was strict. No starches, no dairy, no corn, no wheat, no sugar, no NOTHING! Or at least that's what I felt like. I dropped weight. But I couldn't sustain it. I made it about 69 days. I got down to 211 from 225. The weight would come back. It came back hard too. Now, I was up to 239.

I turned 37 in August of 2016. As I was sitting at the kitchen table with my family, I wasn't happy. I was fat and out of shape. My mindset had not been right. As I looked at my beautiful wife and my handsome son I thought to myself, "I don't know how I'm going to be able to turn this around."

The only goal I had accomplished up to that point in 2016 was eating a two-pound donut. Grief. Talk about underachieving.

Chapter Eight: Two Days in One

"I want to start working out at 5 a.m. each morning."

That's what my great friend Luke mentioned to me one day. We both needed to get in shape. Luke's work schedule meant that he had to work out early in the morning. When he told me he wanted to meet up at 5 a.m. at the gym, I thought he was nuts. I was typically waking up at 5 or 5:30. This meant that I would have to wake up at 4 a.m. so I could get to the gym on time. No way I could do it.

But I wanted to help him. So I did. We both needed one another. While the first few weeks were brutal, there was something else that was taking place, even though I didn't know it. I was setting myself up for future success. I was priming the pump to write this book eventually, and I didn't realize it. I recognized that there were some things off in my life. My wife had experienced what's called a molar pregnancy the year before. We were heartbroken that we wouldn't be having a second child.

To make matters worse, my wife required chemotherapy (she did not have cancer). We began going to M.D. Anderson in Houston. The strongest people ARE NOT in the health club bench pressing and squatting. The strongest people ARE FOUND in places like M.D. Anderson. The employees have to be strong to assist others every day who suffer from a life-threatening disease. The families of the patients have to be strong as they see their loved ones going through so much. But the patients are the strongest! They never quit! Going to M.D. Anderson was a game changer. My wife didn't have cancer, but as part of the protocol for the molar pregnancy, and because her HCG (hormone) levels were not returning back to normal, this was required. I learned a lot about gratitude through all of the visits we made. I learned how strong my wife really is. So did she. That experience changed so much for us, both good and bad. We indeed were thankful Nikki didn't have cancer. The ordeal, however, put a strain on our marriage and our pocketbook.

So how did waking up at 4 a.m. each morning set me up for future success? It showed me that I could live two days in one. Yep, that's right. Like so many people, I had started a lot of things, like reading books, only to stop midway. I was like the man that Jesus mentioned in Luke 14:28-29 who began to build but never finished. I used the same ole excuse that so many uses…"I DON'T HAVE TIME…" That's false. I have plenty of time, and so do you. We get to decide. This will become important to fully grasp and appreciate as we work on going beyond the scale. You have plenty of time to exercise, to eat healthily, and to change your mindset. We get to decide. I decided that change needed to take place immediately.

Waking up at 4 a.m. was precisely what I needed. My body eventually began to adapt. I started reading and finishing more books. I read a book about the best sleeping habits called *Power Sleep: The Revolutionary Program That Prepares Your Mind For Peak Performance* by Dr. James B. Maas. I read books about thinking positively. Reading is fundamental. I began doing mental exercises. Every morning I took the opportunity to start to rewire my brain. I focused on things that were positive. I began to pray more to God. I would write out phrases from the Scriptures over and over and over. I would write out daily affirmations hundreds of times. Waking up so early began to allow me to live two days in one.

It was amazing. It still is. I haven't stopped. Why would I? It is almost like a secret weapon. So many people talk about the benefit of waking up early, but many still throw out excuses. If you want something, you may need to do something different. Give it a shot. Wake up earlier in the day. I had more time to read my Bible without feeling pressured or rushed. I had more time to really talk to God, and not just mumble some quick prayer to Him. I will tell you if the only time you're praying to God is when there is food in front of you, there's something wrong. I needed time alone with God to change my mindset. So do you. Now I know what you're thinking, "There's no way I can wake up so early. Sounds like a good idea, but it won't work for me." Oh really? Let me ask you a couple of questions.

- How do you know you can't wake up this early?
- If it were to help you accomplish more of your goals, would you do it?

The problem so many people have is that they limit themselves. They have weak beliefs about themselves and what they can really do. These false beliefs often get in the way of powerful change and growth. Many struggle with what I call the grasshopper effect. Are you familiar with the grasshopper effect? I'm sure you are, but you just have never heard of described in this way. In the Old Testament in Numbers 13, the Israelites were told to take the land of Canaan. But after spying on the land, 10 of the 12 spies came back with a negative report. They convinced the people to think they couldn't do it.

They described themselves as mere grasshoppers compared to the people in the land. Do you know what happened? They were not able to do it. They held these limiting beliefs, and those beliefs became a reality. They didn't focus on how BIG GOD IS. Instead, they allowed the F.U.D. factor (something I got from a friend of mine) to settle in their minds. The F.U.D. factor stands for Fear, Uncertainty, and Doubt.

Fear delayed an entire nation from accomplishing their goal. The battle was already won. Will the same happen to you? Do you really think you couldn't wake up early if that's what it took to accomplish your goals? Part of what we will need to do to go beyond the scale is to eliminate fear, uncertainty, and doubt. We will also have to be willing to sacrifice. I had to sacrifice a few things to wake up at 4 a.m. each morning. Those sacrifices were worth it. The biggest thing I let go of was watching television. There's really nothing good on television. Watching the news will make you scared. I get tired of watching football players hurting themselves. This is one of the simplest things you can do to gain more time in your life. I even let go of ESPN (this was huge) and watching sporting events.

I've stopped watching the NBA playoffs and Finals. I've passed the baton on watching the Olympics. What about the World Series? Nope. What about the Super Bowl? Okay, I'm a little bit of hypocrite with football because I will watch some of that game. Here's what I've learned: If you want something then you have to make sacrifices. Maybe the word "sacrifice" isn't the proper word to use. The more I let go of stuff that was stealing my time, the more my eyes were open to how much I could truly accomplish. I can achieve anything if I'm willing to put in the work. I was now living two days in one. I finished reading a 500 page in a few weeks. As I prayed, my prayers got bigger. I was training my sub-conscious. I'm convinced this time in the morning, was what I needed, for me to make lasting changes both physically and spiritually. Do you know what happened? Change happened. It was now time for me to go beyond the scale. I put myself in the right position to succeed by waking up early. But I still need some help. Help would come in the form of an email.

Chapter Nine: One Year of Focus

"Dreams really do come true."

I believe it was in July of 2016 when I wrote something like the quote above in one of my journals. I was doing a fun exercise where you are to write down 10 things you would love to experience. One of the things that I wrote down was about to come true. I wanted to work out with a certain health and fitness coach. That dream would become a reality.

In August of 2016, I got an email from that particular health and fitness coach. This one was different. I was sitting at the kitchen table. On my screen, I read about a great opportunity of being able to work out with him via Facebook. I was ready to sign up. But there was a problem. It was through Facebook, and I had deactivated my account earlier that year. I read a book called "Deep Work" by Cal Newport that convinced me to get off social media. I decided to unplug from the Matrix. I went underground. But now this opportunity was at the tip of my fingers. I desperately needed help. So I did it. I plugged back into the Matrix. I signed up again to Facebook. I had zero friends. The only reason why I did it was to be able to join this program.

As I began the four-week program, I weighed 239 pounds. My waist was about 40 inches. I was able to experience positive peer pressure from the workout team. I was going to make the best of those four weeks. We worked on nutrition, exercise routine, and mindset. I remember at the beginning of the program as we talked about goals, I decided to set up a photo shoot. I was going to give myself 12 weeks to transform my body. I had said those kinds of words to myself many times before. But this time was different! Here's why. I followed through. I picked up the phone and set up the photo shoot. I promise you after I hung up the phone I felt a massive surge of energy. There was a switch that was flipped in my mind. What was it? It was BELIEF! For the first time in a long time, I believed I would genuinely change my body and mind. I will never forget that feeling. It was unbelievable.

When we truly believe we can do something, then watch out world. Get ready to see your dreams come true! This is what was about to take place for me.

In September I wrote some more of this book you're reading without even knowing it. I had my own BEYOND THE SCALE moment. Let me explain. One of the things I kept hearing from my online coach was that we should weigh once a month. Could that be right? So many people weigh themselves once a day. This is what I had done in the past. Once a week didn't sound too bad, but not once a month? How in the world was I ever going to be able only to weigh myself once a MONTH? I didn't initially buy into that philosophy. But as the days continued I began to see the WHY behind it. When you understand the WHY, then you will have more CLARITY. It wasn't merely about the scale. There were other ways to measure our success.

Another breakthrough moment happened to me, which helped me to go beyond the scale. I ended up throwing both of my scales away. I even made a video of it. It was a game changer. This is why I asked you to throw your scale or scales away. I didn't need them. Little did I know that decision would help me reach this point. I was free, and I didn't realize it. As those four weeks continued, I began to see there was so much more for me to focus on rather than the scale. I could focus on how often I was eating healthy meals. I could focus on whether or not I was pushing myself in the workouts. I could focus on encouraging others who were on the same journey as I was. It was working. Those four weeks flew by fast. The journey would continue for a year. I would eventually be able to meet my coach in person. Then something else happened. He asked me if I could speak and talk about faith and fitness. I was honored to speak. I called the talk, "Faith, Family, Fitness, Food." This would eventually become my platform on my blog. Many of the things I've already mentioned were discussed in the presentation I gave. The motivational speech went well. I was asked to speak in April. I called that talk "Beyond the Scale." Many of the ideas of this book came from the presentation I gave.

Chapter Ten: The Motivator Is in Da House!

"I was talking to my mom on the phone... and I told her that the motivator was here."

Those were the words one of the employees at my local gym said to me on Sunday, May 14, 2017. I was leaving the gym. I had a great session of H.I.I.T (High Interval Intensity Training) on the treadmill. As I was leaving the gym, I said goodbye to her. She asked me how my workout was. I responded by saying it was good. I told her I like to have fun with my workouts. I felt compelled to say that because that morning, and pretty much every other time I work out I am the weird guy at the gym yelling and screaming while exercising. What's even scarier is when I sing while I run. It's not a good thing to hear. But she said something, which stuck with me. She said, "I was talking to my mom on the phone. She lives in Alabama. I told her the motivator was here." At first, I didn't know what she was talking about until I realized she was talking about me. Wow. What a compliment.

This wasn't the only time I heard something like this. The week before there was a couple at the gym running on the treadmills next to me. I was doing the same thing as I do every workout. I was sweaty, loud, and fired up. I always wonder what people think of me when I'm yelling and screaming. I'm pretty sure some of them are laughing at me. But who cares, right? I knew what the couple was thinking because they told me. The woman told me to "Keep Going! What you are doing and saying is motivating us." Again, I was shocked.

Something was being confirmed to me. I can motivate and inspire others. I'm not trying to sound cocky here. For a while, this was something I didn't necessarily accept. But the more I reflect and consider all that has happened, I have come to embrace the fact I can motivate others.

One of the great benefits of the fitness journey I was on was how I was losing weight and getting stronger. My confidence was increasing. I believed more I would be successful. It was happening right before my eyes. Yet something else was beginning to emerge. I started to fall in love with writing. I make no claims of being some prolific author or writer. But I've been writing for a long time. As a preacher, I've been writing sermons for almost a decade. I'm writing sermons, short blogs, or workbooks. I believe all of the writing has helped me to get to this point now, and I didn't even know it. This is another reason why I love the early morning hours because it allows me the opportunity to write. The exercise I was also doing was unleashing so many ideas and thoughts I didn't know I had. During my transformation beginning back in August of 2016, was when I really started to enjoy writing. Many of the ideas of this book occurred during those days. In 2017, I also joined another group called B.L.A.S.T. (www.blastmentoring.com) by Shannon Ethridge. BLAST stands for "Building leaders, authors, speakers, and teachers." Shannon gave me a great deal of motivation to begin my blog and eventually a website. She continues to be a great source of encouragement and support. As a result of my transformation and taking this writing course I began creating. I began first by writing a short book about my father "Live and learn or Learn and live: A short book for young boys without fathers" that's available on Amazon. Then I created my first coloring book. I got the idea of a coloring book from listening to a former student that was part of the BLAST program. She had created a coloring book. I had never really been into coloring books, but the concept of creating a coloring book was interesting. I wondered if I could do the same thing. And if I was going to create a book, what it would look like? It had to be something connected to my life. Then it hit me. I had been journaling for months. I had been writing out motivational phrases to myself over and over. I didn't think people would want to do the same thing (I would write the same phrase 20-30 times). But what if they could color these motivational phrases? What if I created a coloring book full of motivational thoughts from A-Z? That's what I did. I got the A-Z idea from my preacher back in Rockford Illinois. He would use ABC's in his sermons sometimes to make a point. I loved them. I began to do the same thing when I was in Columbia Missouri. I love doing it. I don't know if the brethren did. So this is where the idea for my first coloring came from. During this time I read a book by James Altoucher called *Choose Yourself*. I learned in this book about Create Space. This is a website affiliated with Amazon. It allows people to publish books. So I created my first coloring book. It's called *Color Your Way To Success*. It was fun putting it together. I was nervous about what others would say. But who cares, right? I couldn't let fear hold me back. So I wrote it. Guess what? People bought it and liked it. Seeing success from that book, I decided to create another one. This coloring book was also personal. I called it *Color Your Way Through Chemo*. My motivation for this came from seeing what my wife experienced. This was another coloring book that goes from A–Z and is filled with motivational phrases for those who have to take chemo. It's designed to give them strength as they battle through a tough condition. Well, now I couldn't stop creating. I made a Chemo coloring book for kids, which goes from A–Z, but is a mixture of motivational phrases and animals. Then I created a fourth book called, *Color Your Way To Releasing The Weight*. The same concept except I added more thoughts as you color. I then shifted and created a motivational journal called "Faith, Family, Fitness, Food: A 31 day motivational journal." I learned the importance of journaling during my transformation. I wanted to create a journal that would compliment what I was already doing in my morning routine. So I did. This journal has…

- 31 days of motivational thoughts from me.
- A place for one to write out their prayers.
- A place to make a gratitude list.
- Space to write out what you're going to eat and actually ate.
- What you did well nutrition wise.
- A motivational thought to write to yourself.
- Finally, a place to write down what you're going to do for exercise.

As I write this I've noticed I haven't even told you how much weight I lost. It's because when it comes to genuinely transforming our lives, it's not about the scale. It's about the journey, belief, relationships, and changing others for good. I did, however, experience a change on the scale. I released 20 pounds in those first 12 weeks. Yes. Success. Victorious. From November 20-December 29th I released an additional six pounds. Never in my life had I released weight during Thanksgiving and Christmas. That just doesn't happen. But it did for me. During the holiday season of 2017, I was able to wear all of my clothes including the BROWN SUIT! YES. Releasing the weight is possible. It's possible to keep the weight off. You can do it. But it will require that you go BEYOND THE SCALE.

I've learned that I'm able to motivate others and I'm also able to motivate myself. We have to be able to motivate ourselves. In this physical and spiritual journey, there will be times when you will have to travel alone. You will not always have others cheering you on. In fact, you will outgrow others with respect to accomplishments, mindset, and determination. The same motivation people gave you one year, may no longer be the motivation you need to get to the next level. You will have to continue to go beyond the scale. You will have to go beyond your past success.

Chapter Eleven: You Are Not a Three Digit Number

"The scale does not define your worth!"

What defines your worth is the fact that you were created in the image of God. When you open up the word of God, we read in <u>Genesis 1:26</u>, that we are made in the image of God. This is what makes us valuable. This is what makes us unique. Yet many allow themselves to be defined by the scale. Quit weighing yourself down with what the dreaded scale may say.

I recognize that the scale has its place for being a tool to measure where we are in our weight loss journey. Yet too many use it as the only tool, the final judge that determines whether they have succeeded or failed. That's going to STOP RIGHT NOW! We are so fixated on the number of the scale. There are a couple of problems when we focus too much on the scale. First, when all of our attention is on how much we weigh we will become short-sighted. We blind ourselves to the bigger picture of what we are trying to accomplish. When we want to lose weight, there's typically a more significant reason than just the number.

- Maybe we've been recently diagnosed with a health condition that has scared us, and we realize we have to make some changes immediately.
- Maybe you've seen someone suffering physically, and you realize you need to take control of your life. It could be your children and seeing those precious faces looking up at you every day, and you realizing you need to be around for them.
- Maybe it's because of your faith in God. You know He wants you to be a good steward of how you take care of your body.
- Some people may be looking for validation of self-worth because of poor relationships with mom and/or dad growing up.

There's typically always something bigger behind why people want to lose weight. Even if people say, "I want to lose weight so I can look good..." there is still something behind those thoughts. People want approval. People want to feel worthy. There's always something bigger than just the three-digit number. People want to feel better physically.

But if all we do is focus solely on a number, we will become short-sighted. We will miss the big picture, our WHY, and ultimately will fall short. I think this is why so many can make significant changes in 12 weeks, only to gain it all back. I speak from experience. They were solely focused on short-term success. They were too concerned about the number on the scale. They failed to see the big picture that it's not about the scale. There's something else people often fail to see. Many fail to recognize how we are more than flesh and blood. We are spirit beings. Remember Genesis 1:26? Listen to what the Prophet Moses wrote concerning what God said in the beginning…

> Then God said, "Let us make man in our image, after our likeness…"

This is why we must go beyond the scale. Our worth and value are based upon the fact that we are spiritual beings. We are more than flesh and blood.

> Some number should never define our WORTH, rather SOMEONE…GOD!

Our value is not based upon our FICO number, bank account number, or the scale. It's based upon how God views us. I am unique, and so are you. We are spirit beings. This is what makes us valuable. Jesus spoke about what is truly valuable. In Luke 9:25 Jesus said,

> "For what does it profit a man if he gains the whole world and loses or forfeits himself?"

Our soul is what's valuable in the eyes of God. I know of grown men who have cried (which men should do) when they genuinely recognize how God sees them. That's because both men and women both struggle with seeing themselves as worth something, much less being valuable. So many people have been hurt in this world. So many struggle with experiencing true love. So many beat themselves up because of the mistakes they have made. That's enough. My friend, say it with me right now…"I am valuable in the eyes of God." I will wait for you to say it.

Did you do it? Good! Now, did you really believe it? I hope you did because it's true. God knows everything about you. He knows the number of hairs on your head. God knows your insecurities. He knows your fears. Now the Lord wants you to know something. He wants you to know that He loves you. God is love, 1 John 4:8. God is love and loves to demonstrate His love.

52

He expressed His love for us in the most significant way possible, John 3:16. He sent His Son Jesus to die for our sins. Everything you need to know about LOVE, HOPE, FORGIVENESS, VALUE, LIFE, REDEMPTION, can be found when you turn and take time to survey the Old Rugged Cross!

If you don't understand WHY you need to go beyond the scale, you will always struggle with the scale. Truly embracing the WHY is the beginning of truly letting go of the scale and the burden it often brings to you. Our goal in life is not to hit a certain number on a scale, but hopefully to LIVE and KNOW the true and LIVING GOD. He can be found if we are willing to seek after Him. This is what the apostle Paul said to the audience in Athens in Acts 17:26-28. Paul said…

"And He made from one man every nation of mankind to live on all the face of the earth, having determined their appointed times and the boundaries of their habitation, that they would seek God, if perhaps they might grope for Him and find Him, though He is not far from each one of us; for in Him we live and move and exist, as even some of your own poets have said, 'For we also are His children.'"

Always remember that you are made in the image of God. Therefore, you are valuable and precious in the sight of God.

What are we really after? What is weight loss and transforming our bodies all about? It's not about the scale but…

- Having the health to be around for our beautiful children.
- Having the strength to be there for a loved one who is battling some disease.
- Having the energy to assist others in need.
- Giving glory to God, by the way, we take care of our bodies.
- About the proper mindset to fight against the devil.
- About being able to see our children get married one day.

Can you see why it's not about the scale? When I first got diagnosed with HCM years ago, I wasn't concerned about the number on the scale. Instead, I was worried about life, and what my condition meant for my family. When my son Joshua was born, I wasn't concerned about the scale. Instead, I was more interested in being in shape, so I can be present to help this precious soul become a man of God.

A friend of mine was recently diagnosed with cancer. What do you think he is really concerned about at this moment? What the scale is telling him, or whether or not he's going to be around for his children in the next five years? Listen very carefully. We have got to get past the scale. There is so much more at stake. Let's start really thinking about what really matters. Let's dive deep into our hearts and tap into what it is that we need to be after. When we do that, we will see that it's not about the scale

Chapter Twelve: The Challenge of Focusing on What Matters

"In two weeks, you can be 20 pounds lighter."

It's statements like these that mess people up. All you have to do is buy something at the grocery store and you will see wild claims like the one mentioned above. Walk into a health club and you will see challenges about losing a lot of weight in a very short period of time. Why are we constantly bombarded with these messages? It's because people are so concerned with the scale.

This is the challenge we must overcome and conquer. We know that we are not just a number. But I would venture to say that almost everyday, we have to struggle with this, at least some of us do. I think inception has taken place for many of us when it comes to the scale. There are some fascinating observations for us to consider when we think about the scale. So many women don't view themselves as beautiful or attractive, because they don't fit the mold that society has constructed for them. There is so much discontent in so many women. Sadly, many husbands don't compliment their wives, as they should. This certainly will not help the self-esteem of these women. This can turn into a vicious cycle for so many women who think that if they can just get to a certain weight, that they will again receive affection from their husband. Husbands, we need to be encouraging our wives with our words, not discouraging them. We need to remind them about their beauty on a regular basis, no matter what the scale says.

If you listen carefully to the conversations of others, you will inevitably hear someone talk about how they need to lose a few more pounds. It's all about the scale number. Even men struggle with this. As men, we are often fighting against our former selves. We remember how much we weighed in college or high school. For some strange reason, we try to recapture those early glory days. But we overlook so much. I have tried to recapture where I was in college. But so much has changed. My body has changed. My mindset has changed. Looking back at that Ben I see someone who was spiritually immature, spiritually flabby, and more concerned about satisfying the lust of the flesh instead of giving glory to God. I was more focused about how my body looked on the outside and in the eyes of others, instead of being concerned about how my soul appeared before God. I remember one time in college my roommate and I had some friends over. One of the girls mentioned to my friend, and me "I would have never thought you two were

Christians." Ouch. But she was right. I was Christian-ish. I spoke about Christianity when it suited me. I talked a good game but my actions were not aligning with my beliefs. When that happens, there will always be conflict. The challenge for us to focus on what it is that really matters.

We put ourselves in this vicious cycle. We often say things like…

"I want to lose just 10 more pounds."

"I've lost of a lot of weight, but I still want to lose more."

"I'm still going after that goal number."

"I want to get my revenge body."

Again, I know that the scale has a role. It is one of many tools that we have at our disposal to see where we are physically. But we can't become so consumed with it, although this is what happens to so many. The bigger challenge for us is to truly focus on what really matters. When I started taking the time to reflect upon my journey I had to really think about a single question. That question was…

"What Is It That Really Matters?"

I don't think I had really thought about this question as much as I should have. For years, I have exercised and tried to eat healthy in vain attempts to look my best. Mirror, Mirror, on the wall, who is the handsomest of them all? ME! Okay, I confess, at times I've been really vain. For many years I was not truly focusing on what really mattered. Maybe this is just a part of getting older. As we get older there are some things in life that just don't matter as much anymore. It no longer matters to me whether or not I watch Sports Center on ESPN. But man, back in the day if I didn't watch Sports Center it was as if the world was coming to and end. It doesn't really matter if I'm not up to date with the latest movies that have been released. It doesn't matter how many suits I have in my closest. It doesn't matter how many friends I have on Facebook. So what is it that really matters? We all need to really think about that question. Does a certain number on the scale really matter so much to you that you will become obsessed to hit it? Does a number on a scale mean so much to you that you will verbally abuse yourself because you haven't successfully hit it? Does a number mean so much to you that you will overlook all of the other successful things have already done?

What really matters to you?

To help you answer this question think about a couple of more questions. Go ahead and write out your answers. Are you ready? Here we go.

If you had a year to live, what would matter to you?

What would you want your children and spouse to say about you at your funeral? I've attached a document at the end of this book where I've written your Eulogy for you. Take some time to read it. Fill in the blanks. I think you will like it. It's what I think we would all like to hear. But what are you doing right now to make all of that possible?

Would you want your children to follow the path you're currently on now?

Where are you with your relationship with God?

Are things becoming a little clearer for you? Answering these questions may help you to think about what is it that should truly matter to you. Now maybe you have read all of this and are still not buying into the concept of going beyond the scale. Maybe, you're saying to yourself, "I just don't know if this is as big of a deal as you are making it." Well then consider this. Have you ever reached your goal weight only to find yourself still not content?

I find this so amazing. For years maybe you've been going after the magical number of 200, or 175, or 135, or 120 pounds. You wake up one sunny morning, stretch out your legs and feet from the bed, crack your toes, walk to the bathroom, and get on the magical scale. Those red or blue digital numbers pop and say, "Congratulations, you have done it." NOW WHAT? Many have had this happened to them and they are still not happy. They still have a spirit of discontentment. Even worse, they may still feel heavy. It's not about the scale. It's not about some number. There's something bigger that's taking place.

Chapter Thirteen: Lay Aside the Other Weight

So what weight do you really need to lose once and for all? What is it that we need to change in our lives so we can get to where we really want to be (and not just some number)? We can be so short-sighted at times with what we really need. Sometimes, we need someone else to help us to see where we are, and what it is that may be holding us back. What weight is holding you back? The extra weight we carry around our bellies, hips, and thighs is often a by-product of something else in our lives that may be amiss. Sometimes the scale is not moving because there's something else that needs to be moved, lifted, or eliminated. Let's consider a couple of thoughts.

Lay Aside the Negative Talk to Yourself

For some of us to go beyond the scale, we are going to have to change our language. Not necessarily the way that we speak to others, but instead how we talk to ourselves. Words are powerful. Words have been able to get nations to go to war. Words have ruined marriages. Words have destroyed local churches. Words from a parent can set their children on a path of success or potential failure. Words are powerful. Think about the Bible. The words in the word can change a person's entire life.

Even how we speak about our transformation can be powerful. Words can shape our mindset for better or for worse. We want to be able to go in the right direction. Therefore, we will need to choose our words carefully.

How do you talk to yourself? Do you speak to yourself the way you talk to others? Are you continually beating yourself up because you failed to be perfect? Newsflash. The only one who lived a perfect life was Jesus. We are going to make mistakes, especially when it comes to laying aside the extra physical weight we may have. But we also need to be sure that we put aside the negative talk we often attack ourselves with. If you keep telling yourself...

"I'm such a failure..."

"I can't seem to get it right..."

"I'm an idiot..."

Then you will never get to where you need to be. Lay aside the weight of negative speech and negatively viewing yourself. Do something else. Change the way you talk about weight loss. Last year I was in Chicago visiting some family. I was talking to my sister about weight loss. During our discussion, she said something powerful. It stuck with me and has caused me to change my language. She mentioned how we often say, "I want to lose..." when it comes to our weight. But something you lose is something that you will eventually find again. When we lose our keys, we go looking for them and will eventually find them. When we lose our cell phone, we are going to look for them quickly and will find them. Sadly, we do the same thing when it comes to our weight. I don't know how much weight I have really lost. Maybe over 100 pounds in my lifetime. That's because I would lose 20 pounds and then later on in the year I would find it again. I kept losing, but I also kept finding. Can you relate? Maybe instead of saying how much weight we want to LOSE, we should change that to how much weight we want to RELEASE. She either made up this idea or got it from someone else. It's not mine. Whoever thought of it, I love it. Changing one word can change everything. Moving forward, whenever you talk about your weight with others change "LOSE" and replace it with "RELEASE."

"I want to RELEASE 20 pounds of fat."

"I have successfully RELEASED 40 pounds in the last year."

"I will continue to RELEASE unwanted fat."

Release that fat once and for all! Don't go looking for it anymore. Say, "I'm never finding this weight again." You will not because you haven't just lost it, you have released it.

Lay aside the weight of harmful speech. Be careful with how you talk to yourself. Be positive. Think about the big picture. Don't give up. And please, give yourself a little credit. Maybe harmful speech is something that you need to lay aside. Before we move on, let's do something. In the space below, write out any negative phrases or thoughts you've had about yourself.

1.

2.

3.

4.

5.

When you see these phrases written out on paper, how do you feel?

Why do you feel like you need to say these negative things to yourself?

Now, let's replace those negative thoughts with things that are positive. In the space below, write out some positive statements to yourself.

1.

2.

3.

4.

5.

Does this make you feel better? It should. You need to believe what you just wrote. But maybe there's something else that may be holding you back from going beyond the scale that you need to lay aside.

Lay Aside the Financial Weight

If there's a weight we do need to lay aside that can hold us back, it could be the burden of financial debt. I'm not going to go into the numbers of the debt crisis, so many are in because you can go on the Internet and quickly find out what the numbers are. If we happen to fall into that category, then we need to take action. The Bible warns us about not becoming shackled with debt, Proverbs 22:7. *"The rich rules over the poor, and the borrower becomes the lender's slave."* Debt produces burdens in our lives. It will cause one to feel heavy, trapped, and overwhelmed. Debt can often be the cause of emotional eating. I've been in debt before, and I absolutely hate it. It

61

can and will bring about fear and worry, which is no way to live. One can be so consumed with trying to get out of debt that they cancel their gym membership, don't make time to exercise, or makes up excuses as to why they can't exercise. It can cause people to grind their teeth at night and not get enough sleep (Ok I'm talking about myself here). It can wreak havoc in a marriage.

Laying aside the weight of financial debt is much like weight loss. It will take time. It's a marathon and not a sprint. We will have to be patient, but make no mistake we will be able to do it. If you struggle with financial debt, then I would suggest that you buy any book written by Dave Ramsey. He will help steer you in the right direction. Before we move on, I want you to do another exercise. I added this after thinking about what a sister in Christ told me in 2017. She had a major shopping problem. She would hide stuff she bought from her husband. She admitted that she was out of control. She also struggles with being overweight. Do you think there is a connection? Maybe there is. Ask yourself a couple of questions.

> Are you seeking validation or self-worth by buying and accumulating stuff?
> Are your finances so out of control that it's having an impact on your health?

If you answer yes to these questions, you will need to spend some time to think about a few things. Maybe trimming down your finances will create a positive ripple effect concerning your health. But perhaps financial debt is not the weight you need to lay aside. Maybe there's another weight that is still making you feel heavy, despite the number on the scale going down.

Lay Aside the Weight of Being an Emotional Hoarder

We need to ask and identify if we are emotional hoarders. Have you ever seen the television show called Hoarders? You can't help but feel bad for those people. They hoard physical stuff in their homes to the point that it ruins their lives. But are we like them? Are we emotional hoarders? Do you know someone like this? Emotions are powerful. God created us with emotions thank goodness. It's normal to feel joy, excitement, fear, anger, loneliness, resentment, and grief. But sometimes we can allow our emotions to dictate how we think and live, which if not careful will become very detrimental. There are countless examples of people in the Bible who were emotional hoarders. They couldn't seem to let go.

For example, take the case of Cain, <u>Genesis 4:3-7</u>. The text says…

"So it came about in the course of time that Cain brought an offering to the LORD of the fruit of the ground. Abel, on his part also brought of the firstlings of his flock and of their fat portions. And the LORD had regard for Abel and for his offering; but for Cain and for his offering He had no regard. So Cain became very angry and his countenance fell. The LORD said to Cain, "Why are you angry? And why has your countenance fallen? If you do well, will not your countenance be lifted up? And if you do not do well, sin is crouching at the door; and its desire is for you, but you must master it."

Cain wasn't happy how God accepted his brother's sacrifice and not his. Cain had no right to be upset with God about this. There was a standard God had given both Cain and Abel, and Cain chose not to give God what He desired. His emotions led him to murder his brother.

What about the descendants of Esau (the Edomites), <u>Genesis 36:1</u>? They harbored bad feelings toward the Israelites. To understand the significance of this, you must understand the relationship between Jacob and Esau. These two were brothers. Esau was the firstborn of Isaac. However, in the process of time, Jacob would take Esau's birthright from him. Esau hated Jacob and desired to kill him. Years would pass, and the anger of Esau diminished. Eventually, he came to love his brother Jacob again. However, the descendants of Esau, the Edomites, would not treat the descendants of Jacob the same way. They would not forgive. They would hold a grudge. They were emotional hoarders, <u>Numbers 20:14-21</u>

From Kadesh Moses then sent messengers to the king of Edom:

"Thus your brother Israel has said, 'You know all the hardship that has befallen us; that our fathers went down to Egypt, and we stayed in Egypt a long time, and the Egyptians treated us and our fathers badly. 'But when we cried out to the LORD, He heard our voice and sent an angel and brought us out from Egypt; now behold, we are at Kadesh, a town on the edge of your territory. 'Please let us pass through your land. We will not pass through field or through vineyard; we will not even drink water from a well.

We will go along the king's highway, not turning to the right or left, until we pass through your territory.'" Edom, however, said to him, "You shall not pass through us, or I will come out with the sword against you."

Due to their hatred toward the Israelites, God would eventually destroy the Edomites. In Malachi 1:1-5 it says,

"The oracle of the word of the LORD to Israel through Malachi. "I have loved you," says the LORD. But you say, "How have You loved us?" Was not Esau Jacob's brother?" declares the LORD. "Yet I have loved Jacob; but I have hated Esau, and I have made his mountains a desolation and appointed his inheritance for the jackals of the wilderness." Though Edom says, "We have been beaten down, but we will return and build up the ruins"; thus says the LORD of hosts, "They may build, but I will tear down; and men will call them the wicked territory, and the people toward whom the LORD is indignant forever."

Being an emotional hoarder will come with consequences. For the Edomites, it came with eternal consequences.

Maybe one of the most prominent examples of someone who was an emotional hoarder was King Saul. Saul would become the first king of Israel. He looked the part as a king, 1 Samuel 9:1-2.

"Now there was a man of Benjamin whose name was Kish the son of Abiel, the son of Zeror, the son of Becorath, the son of Aphiah, the son of a Benjaminite, a mighty man of valor. He had a son whose name was Saul, a choice and handsome man, and there was not a more handsome person than he among the sons of Israel; from his shoulders and up he was taller than any of the people."

The prophet Samuel would anoint Saul to become king over Israel, 1 Samuel 13:1. His rule began well. Yet things quickly changed, 1 Samuel 13:8-14. Saul was not obedient to the Lord. He didn't follow through on the instructions Samuel the prophet gave him. Listen to what happened.

"Now he waited seven days, according to the appointed time set by Samuel, but Samuel did not come to Gilgal; and the people were scattering from him. So Saul said, "Bring to me the burnt offering and the peace offerings." And he offered the burnt offering. As soon as he finished offering the burnt offering, Samuel came; and Saul went out to meet him and to greet him. But Samuel said, "What have you done?" And Saul said, "Because I saw that the people were scattering from me, and that you did not come within the appointed days, and that the Philistines were assembling at Michmash, therefore I said, 'Now the Philistines will come down against me at Gilgal, and I have not asked the favor of the LORD. So I forced myself and offered the burnt offering." Samuel said to Saul, "You have acted foolishly; you have not kept the commandment of the LORD your God, which He commanded you, for now the LORD would have established your kingdom over Israel forever: But now your kingdom shall not endure. The LORD has sought out for Himself a man after is own heart, and the LORD has appointed him as ruler over His people, because you have not kept what the LORD commanded you."

In reality, Saul was a terrible leader. While he looked the part, he didn't lead well. The kingdom would eventually be taken from him as Samuel prophesied. It would be a young man named David that would ultimately replace him. This would not sit well with King Saul. Initially, the relationship between these two men began well. As Saul endured depression, David came to play for him, 1 Samuel 16:14-23.

"Now the Spirit of the LORD departed from Saul, and an evil spirit from the LORD terrorized him. Saul's servants then said to him, "Behold now, an evil spirit from God is terrorizing you. "Let our lord now command your servants who are before you. Let them seek a man who is a skillful player on the harp; and it shall come about when the evil spirit from God is on you, that he shall play the harp with his hand, and you will be well." So Saul said to his servants, "Provide for me now a man who can play well and bring him to me." Then one of the young men said, "Behold, I have seen a son of Jesse the Bethlehemite who is a skillful musician, a mighty man of valor, a warrior, one prudent in speech, and a handsome man; and the LORD is with him." So Saul sent messengers to Jess and said, "Send me your son David who is with the flock." Jesse took a donkey loaded with bread and a jug of wine and a young goat, and sent them to Saul by David his son. Then David came to Saul and attended him; and Saul loved him greatly, and he became his armor bearer. Saul sent to Jesse, saying, "Let David now stand before me, for he has found favor in my sight." So it came about whenever the evil spirit from God came to Saul, David would take the harp and play it with his hand; and Saul would be refreshed and be well, and the evil spirit would depart from him."

But Saul could not control his emotions, 1 Samuel 18:8-9.

"Then Saul became very angry, for this saying displeased him; and he said, "They have ascribed to David ten thousands, but to me they have ascribed thousands. Now what more can he have but the kingdom?" Saul looked at David with suspicion from that day on."

What was it that consumed Saul? Resentment, anger, jealousy, pride, intimidation, deception, and depression consumed his heart, 1 Samuel 18:28-29.

"When Saul saw and knew that the LORD was with David, and that Michal, Saul's daughter, loved him, then Saul was even more afraid of David. Thus Saul was David's enemy continually."

Saul was his worst enemy. He couldn't see how bad he really was, even when others could, 1 Samuel 19:1-5.

"Now Saul told Jonathan his son and all his servants to put David to death. But Jonathan, Saul's son, greatly delighted in David. So Jonathan told David saying, "Saul my father is seeking to put you to death. Now therefore, please be on guard in the morning, and stay in a secret place and hide yourself. "I will go out and stand beside my father in the field where you are, and I will speak with my father about you; if I find out anything, then I will tell you." Then Jonathan spoke well of David to Saul his father and said to him, "Do not let the king sin against his servant David, since he has not sinned against you, and since his deeds have been very beneficial to you. "For he took his life in his hand and struck the Philistine, and the LORD brought about a great deliverance for all Israel; you saw it and rejoiced. Why then will you sin against innocent blood by putting David to death without a cause?"

When others tried to help, he went into defense mode, 1 Samuel 20:30-33.

"Then Saul's anger burned against Jonathan and he said to him, "You son of a perverse, rebellious woman! Do I not know that you are choosing the son of Jesse to your own shame and to the shame of your mother's nakedness? "For as long as the son of Jesse lives on the earth, neither you nor your kingdom will be established. Therefore now, send and bring him to me, for he must surely die." But Jonathan answered Saul his father and said to him, "Why should he be put to death? What has he done?" Then Saul hurled his spear at him to strike him down; so Jonathan knew that his father had decided to put David to death."

His lack of self-control and obsession with David hurt others, 1 Samuel 22:17.

"And the king said to the guards who were attending him, "Turn around and put the priests of the LORD to death, because their hand also is with David and because they knew that he was fleeing and did not reveal it to me." But the servants of the king were not willing to put forth their hands to attack the priests of the LORD."

His story would not end well, 1 Samuel 31:1-4.

"Now the Philistines were fighting against Israel, and the men of Israel fled from before the Philistines and fell slain on Mount Gilboa. The Philistines overtook Saul and his sons; and the Philistines killed Jonathan and Abinadab and Malchi-shua the sons of Saul. The battle went heavily against Saul, and the archers hit him; and he was badly wounded by the archers. Then Saul said to his armor bearer, "Draw your sword and pierce me through with it, otherwise these uncircumcised will come and pierce me through and make sport of me." But his armor bearer would not, for he was greatly afraid. So Saul took his sword and fell on it."

Saul couldn't let go. He played the role of a victim, even though David had done nothing against him. He was an emotional hoarder. How we go about controlling our emotions, harboring resentment, anger, bitterness, etc. will have a direct impact when it comes to making the necessary changes that we may need to make. While these are cases of individuals who were emotional hoarders, and who got in their own way, I want you to think about someone who was not an emotional hoarder. I want to go back to the young man David we just discussed. David would eventually replace Saul as king over Israel. While David and Saul's life intertwined, the two men couldn't have been more different. Saul was wicked while David was righteous. David could have retaliated.

David had more cause to be upset than Saul had. And we find that's not how David responded. David did what was right, even when he could have been fueled with revenge, 1 Samuel 24:4-10.

The men of David said to him, "Behold, this is the day of which the LORD said to you, 'Behold; I am about to give your enemy into your hand, and you shall do to him as it seems good to you.'" Then David arose and cut off the edge of Saul's robe secretly. It came about afterward that David's conscience bothered him because he had cut off the edge of Saul's robe. So he said to his men, "Far be it from me because of the LORD that I should do this thing to my lord, the LORD's anointed, to stretch out my hand against him, since he is the LORD's anointed." David persuaded his men with these words and did not allow them to rise up against Saul. And Saul arose, left the cave, and went on his way. Now afterward David arose and went out of the cave and called after Saul, saying, "My lord the king!" And when Saul looked behind him, David bowed with his face to the ground and prostrated himself. David said to Saul, "Why do you listen to the words of men, saying, 'Behold, David seeks to harm you'? "Behold, this day your eyes have seen that the LORD had given you today into my hand in the cave, and some said to kill you, but my eye had pity on you; and I said, 'I will not stretch out my hand against my lord, for he is the LORD's anointed.' "Now, my father, see! Indeed, see the edge of your robe in my hand! For in that I cut off the edge of your robe and did not kill you, know and perceive that there is no evil or rebellion in my hands, and I have not sinned against you, though you are lying in wait for my life to take it."

David was truly a man after God's own heart. He did what was right. He controlled his emotions. Are we following in the path of Saul or David? What we hold on to in life is powerful.

How was David able to avoid becoming an emotional hoarder like Saul?

First, David feared God. Vengeance belongs to God, not men, 1 Samuel 26:10. David also said, "As the LORD lives, surely the LORD will strike him, or his day will come that he dies, or he will go down into battle and perish." David was right.

Second, David controlled himself and didn't allow Saul to dictate his emotions.

Third, David had a spirit of peace where he attempted to find common ground with Saul, 1 Samuel 26:18. He also said, "Why then is my lord pursuing his servant? For what have I done? Or what evil is in my hand?

Fourth, David refused to harbor ill will toward Saul, 2 Samuel 1:17. *Then David chanted with this lament over Saul and Jonathan his son.* He wrote a song of lament for both Saul and Jonathan.

Fifth, David valued his life, 1 Samuel 26:24. He wanted the feud between him and Saul to end. To live in the past and harbor resentment toward Saul would freeze his progression in life. David refused to become an emotional hoarder.

Now, what about us? When it comes to controlling our emotions, are we more like Saul or David?

- Are we emotional hoarders? Do we harbor resentment or revenge in our hearts? Are we unwilling to forgive certain people? If so, then we have some problems to address.
- Being an emotional hoarder is no way to live. All it will do is consume our lives, disrupt unity among God's people, hinder our influence in the world, hurt others, and potentially cause us to lose our souls. That's not what we have been called to be. I recognize I don't know what you may have been through in your life. We all have a story to tell. Many have some kind of traumatic event they have experienced. Yet, becoming an emotional hoarder is the not right thing to do. In the long run, we will only hurt ourselves. We will hold ourselves back from the transformation (physically and spiritually) we need. But as I type this, I also recognize how this is easier said than done. In the past, I've struggled with anger issues. I've struggled with processing events and emotions I've had from the past. It indeed is a process. But with the help of the Lord, with assistance from brethren, and with even some professional guidance we can do it.

The scriptures provide us with how we can overcome some of the emotional challenges we may face. There are some thoughts and passages we need to remember.

Know the power of God, Romans 1:16.

a. *For I am not ashamed of the gospel, for it is the power of God for salvation to everyone who believes, to the Jew first and also to the Greek.*

b. The gospel of Jesus has the power to save. It has the power to change lives. Know that it's possible for us to improve. The apostle Paul was able to change after learning of the resurrection of Jesus, Acts 9:26-27. *When he came to Jerusalem, he was trying to associate with the disciples; but they were all afraid of him, not believing that he was a disciple. But Barnabas took hold of him and brought him to the apostles and described to them how he had seen the Lord on the road, and that He had talked to him, and how at Damascus he had spoken out boldly in the name of Jesus.* The gospel has the power to change our hearts as well. Do we believe that God can change us? We should.

c.   We must practice self-control, <u>Galatians 5:22</u>. *"But the fruit of the Spirit is love, joy, peace, patience, kindness, goodness, faithfulness, gentleness, self-control; against such things there is no law."* This includes our emotions. Self-control is more than just what we put in our mouths. It's more than just ensuring that we get to the gym a certain number of times each week. Self-control is also about controlling our thoughts, our emotions, and our actions. God has given us feelings. In no way am I saying we should live our lives without expressing any emotions. That would be silly and unhealthy. But we must control them.

We must forgive others as God has forgiven us, <u>Colossians 3:13</u>. *"...Bearing with one another, and forgiving each other, whoever has a complaint against anyone; just as the Lord forgave you, so also should you."* This can be hard to do. It was hard to forgive my father for what he did to my mother and my family. Yet it was something that I needed to do. We desire that people forgive us when we fall short. We must be willing to do the same for others. It was Jesus who said in <u>Luke 6:36</u>, *"Be merciful, just as your Father is merciful."* Like our Savior and like our Father in heaven, we need to be willing to forgive as they have forgiven us.

We need to admit, express, process, and seek to resolve our feelings. This has been a hard one for me. On the one hand, I recognize that emotions are normal. On the other hand, I also understand how easy it can suppress our emotions when we should really allow ourselves to feel them and process them. It's okay to say that we are angry. In fact, in <u>Ephesians 4:26</u> the Holy Spirit says, *"Be angry..."* He also says a lot more about what we are to do with our anger. The Spirit of truth also reminds us to "Be angry, and yet do not sin..." That's the challenging part. I think there's something here for us to unpack and dive into. Anger can cause us to do a lot of things. I know my father had a lot of anger issues. He came from a broken home. There were a lot of family issues that he had to endure. I honestly think (we never got a chance to talk about all of this) my father didn't know how to process his anger. As a result, it led him to alcoholism. It was always interesting to see how my father was only able to cry when he was drunk. Now again, I could be wrong about this because I wasn't around him all the time, but from my observation, he was able to express his emotions more when he was under the influence. As a child, I also struggled with anger issues. Some of that may have been due to growing up with a parent who was an alcoholic. I've struggled at times with expressing my emotions and allowing myself to process and admit how I may feel. Yet this is something that we must do. When it comes to emotions like anger, it's okay to be angry. But let's remember what else the Holy Spirit said in Ephesians 4:26.

a. *"Be angry..."* It's okay for us to become angry. It's normal. We are made in the image of God, Genesis 1:26. Some may be surprised that God can become angry. In Psalm 7:11, it says, *God is a righteous judge, and a God who has indignation every day.* His anger is justified and motivated by love. God is angry over sinful behavior and lack of repentance. This should strike fear in us. It should also help us to see that it's okay to be angry. Jesus was angry when He witnessed the sinful behavior taking place in the temple, John 2:13-17. The text says, *The Passover of the Jews was near, and Jesus went up to Jerusalem. And He found in the temple those who were selling oxen and sheep and doves, and the money changers seated at their tables. And He made a scourge of cords, and drove them all out of the temple, with the sheep and the oxen; and He poured out the coins of the money changers and overturned their tables; and to those who were selling the doves He said, "Take these things away; stop making My Father's house a place of business." His disciples remembered that it was written, "ZEAL FOR YOUR HOUSE WILL CONSUME ME."* He had every right to be angry. It's okay for us to become angry. What's not okay for us to do is to lie about our anger. A preacher once said, "It's not a sin to be angry, but it is a sin to lie about it." How true. I think we may struggle with being honest with ourselves at times about our emotions. Being angry is okay. But there's more.

b. *"And yet do not sin..."* It's okay to be angry, yet God expects us to control our emotions. This is where the challenge often is. It's sometimes challenging for us not to cross that line when our anger becomes sinful. I think some of the previous examples of Cain and the Edomites provide us with some examples of what that may look like when we can cross the line and sin. As we deal with our emotions, it's important to remember who we are as children of God. We are new creatures in Christ. We must recognize that the Holy Spirit is watching us according to Ephesians 4:30. We must realize that nothing good will result from allowing our emotions to get out of control. It will only bring devastation. While one can use anger as fuel to prove others wrong and to accomplish certain things in life, anger will only take you so far. When we hold on to anger, we will be the ones who will ultimately be hurt. Nothing good will happen when a spouse is so angry with their mate they retaliate physically, hold a grudge, allow bitterness to consume them, and reach the point of hating that person. Yet I've seen it happen far too often. It's a danger for me, and it's a danger for you. This is why we must remember what else is said in Ephesians 4:26.

c. *"Do not let the sun go down on your anger…"* The Holy Spirit wants us to take action. He doesn't want things to sit, to fester, to grow, and to become worse. This part of the passage is tough, but it something that we must do. Having a crucial conversation instead of allowing our emotions to consume is tough. But this is what we must do. We need to know reconciliation is possible. If Esau and Jacob could hug, cry, and continue their relationship, it's possible for us to overcome anger.

d. *"And do not give the devil an opportunity…"* When we fail to listen to the words of the Holy Spirit, we open the door to the devil. He is the real enemy according to 1 Peter 5:8. He is motivated by anger and hatred. He would love for us to follow in his footsteps. He got Cain. He got Saul. He got the Edomites. What about us? Will we allow the devil an opportunity to consume our hearts? We must decide if we want to be like the devil or like our heavenly Father. The devil is motivated by anger. God is not. God is full of compassion, mercy, and forgiveness. The devil doesn't want us to resolve a matter, but rather tear down and devour. God wants us to forgive and reconcile. We have a choice. We get to decide what our hearts will look like. Anger is an emotion that we will all experience. It's an emotion we can control. It's one that will have deadly consequences if we don't manage it. It could be why you haven't enjoyed the success you've wanted both physically, spiritually, and emotionally. Are you holding on to anger? It's time to clean house. It's time to let it go. Our goal is to be imitators of God, Ephesians 5:1. Be angry and yet do not sin.

We must strive for peace and unity. I don't know what was going on with Euodia and Syntyche in Philippians 4:2. But it needed to be resolved. They were to live in harmony. When it comes to holding on to certain emotions, we will have to seek peace and unity. We will have to figure out what's happening and strive to fix and resolve those matters. Being an emotional hoarder will hinder the success we seek.

Finally, we must leave all things in God's hands, 2 Timothy 4:14. The apostle Paul is an excellent example of how we ultimately have to trust in the Lord. Alexander, the coppersmith, harmed Paul. I don't know precisely in what way. Notice however how Paul said God would repay him. Paul could have allowed anger and bitterness to consume him. But I don't believe that he did. There was too much at stake. He did know one thing. God would repay Alexander. Wow. What a man of great faith and strength. Being able not to allow emotions to consume you demonstrates great power. That's what we must strive to live every day.

When things get out of whack in our lives, we tend to run to food. Food is such a great friend. We must recognize however that food is going to let us down. After we come down from the sugar high, we will still have to face reality. The challenge is that we need food to survive, John 6:5.

> **Therefore Jesus, lifting up His eyes and seeing that a large crowd was coming to Him, said to Philip, "Where are we to buy bread, so that these may eat?"**

Food is a blessing from God and is to be enjoyed. Solomon said,

> **"I know that there is nothing better for them than to rejoice and to do good in one's lifetime; moreover, that every man**

who eats and drinks sees good in all his labor-it is the gift of God", Ecclesiastes 3:12-13.

But instead of continually running to food, we need to be running more to God, His word, and time with Him in prayer. When a man named Nehemiah in the Old Testament received terrible news, observe below how he responded, Nehemiah 1:1-4.

"The words of Nehemiah the son of Hacaliah. Now it happened in the month Chislev, in the twentieth year, while I was in Susa the capitol, that Hanani, one of my brothers, and some men from Judah came; and I asked them concerning the Jews who had escaped and had survived the captivity, and about Jerusalem. They said to me, "The remnant there in the province who survived the captivity are in great distress and reproach, and the wall of Jerusalem is broken down and its gates are burned with fire." When I heard these words, I sat down and wept and mourned for days; and I was fasting and praying before God of heaven."

He could eat later. He needed something more powerful. He needed the hand of God.

The truth is only God can truly satisfy us, Psalm 90:14. Here the Psalmist says...

"Satisfy us in the morning with your steadfast love, that we may rejoice and be glad all our days..."

True satisfaction will only come from God. We have to believe that because it's true.

If you have watched the television show called Hoarders, I'm sure you have thought, "Why live that way?" That's what we need to be thinking about when it comes to our hearts. Are you an emotional hoarder? Is something from the past holding you down from living the life God wants you to have? When do you think you should release those feelings? How will you feel when you release those emotions once and for all? Write down your thoughts below.

_____

_____

_____

_____

_____

_____

_____

_____

_____

_____

Lay Aside the Weight of Sin

Yet, there's another weight that could truly be holding us back. It's not 3 digits, but rather 3 letters. It's rarely discussed, but we all know it. We've all have done it. It will often torment us and overwhelm us with guilt, until it is resolved. I'm talking about SIN.

Sin is real! The Holy Spirit helps us to understand this. Do you have a Bible? Look up <u>Romans 3:23</u> and write out what it says here:

_____

Sadly some preachers ignore teaching about sin. Sadly, some who profess to be Christians don't want to talk about this either. That's really odd when you consider the fact that Jesus said so much about it. If you don't believe me take a look inside of the Bible and see what He said. Okay, I'm going to give you a homework assignment. I'm going to give you some Bible verses. I want you to open your Bible, read them, and write them out. What does Jesus say? Read...

- John 8:24:

_____

- John 5:14:

_____

_____

_____

- Mark 2:9-10:

_____

_____

_____

What did you learn? What did Jesus say? There are many other passages that we could consider. My point is simple. Sin is a big problem. It's a weight that we all need to address, yet so few do. Could this be the weight that is holding you down? Is this the weight you truly need to lay aside? You can have your six-pack, thick quad muscles, and bulging biceps, but if you haven't addressed the problem of sin, you will always be heavy and weak. We need a spotter when it comes to our sins. No wait, we need a SAVIOR! That SAVIOR is Jesus! We need to SPRINT to Him. He came to deliver us from our sins. Jesus came from a poor family from the dusty streets of Nazareth. He was a carpenter. But He was more than just a man. He is the Son of God who came to take away the sin of the world. That's what John the Baptist said of Him in John 1:29. How did John the Baptist describe Jesus in this verse? Write the verse below.

_____

No one else could do what Jesus did. The great prophet Moses couldn't. The strong man named Samson couldn't. The wisest man to live named Solomon couldn't solve the problem of sin. No amount of animal sacrifices could do it.

Jesus is the ultimate fighter. He is the ultimate weightlifter. The Mr. Universe award is not big enough for Him, because He created the Universe, John 1:1-4,14. Notice what the scripture says.

"In the beginning was the Word, and the Word was with God, and the Word was God. He was in the beginning with God. All things came into being through Him, and apart from Him nothing came into being that has come into being. In Him was life, and the life was the Light of men. And the Word became flesh, and dwelt among us, and we saw His glory, glory as of the only begotten from the Father, full of grace and truth."

He would die on the cross for our sins. We get tired doing the Iron Cross with some light dumbbells, but Jesus endured the Old Rugged Cross. What held Him on the cross, as one man said was not three nails, but rather a four-letter word LOVE! He died for the sins of the world. The debt He paid for us was massive. So debt was so much that as He died on the cross, it became dark for 3 hours, Matthew 27:45.

"Now from the sixth-hour darkness fell upon all the land until the ninth hour."

He was the only one that was cross fit. The debt of our sin was so heavy that Jesus cried out to the Father, Matthew 27:46.

About the ninth hour, Jesus cried out with a loud voice, saying, "Eli, Eli, LAMA SABACHTHANI?" that is, "MY GOD, MY GOD, WHY HAVE YOU FORSAKEN ME?"

The guiltless paid the ransom fee for the guilty! That's love. That's sacrifice. It could be that so many have a hard time going beyond the scale because they are so weighed down from their sins. Salvation in Christ is a free gift that is offered to all.

"For the wages of sin is death, but the free gift of God is eternal life in Christ Jesus our Lord", Romans 6:23.

"Come to Me, all who are weary and heavy-laden, and I will give you rest. Take My yoke upon you and learn from Me, for I am gentle and humble in heart, and YOU WILL FIND REST FOR YOUR SOULS. For My yoke is easy and My burden is light." Matthew 11:28

Salvation is found in Jesus. Through His blood that was shed on the cross, we can find deliverance from our sins, Ephesians 1:7-8.

"In Him, we have redemption through His blood, the forgiveness of our trespasses, according to the riches of His grace which He lavished on us..."

You can receive God's amazing grace when you follow the detailed instructions and listen to Jesus, Luke 13:3; Mark 16:16.

"I tell you, no, but unless you repent, you will all likewise perish."

"He who has believed and has been baptized shall be saved; but he who has disbelieved shall be condemned."

The scale is NOTHING! Three digits will never define you or me! Our worth is found in God. It's time for us to go beyond the scale. Leave the past in the past. Go to the one who can change your life inside and out. There's nothing worse than having a guilty conscious. There's nothing heavier than feeling like you have no hope to continue. A man described as the Philippian Jailer in Acts 16:25-34 felt like his life had reached a point of no hope. Two men of God were in prison but not because of any wrongdoing. But God moved. Around midnight as these two men sang praises to God, an earthquake occurred. Everyone in the prison cells had the opportunity to escape. This would have spelled doom for the jailer because his job was to make sure that no one escaped. If they did, his life would be over. As the jailer saw what happened, he felt like he had only two options. He could stick around and face punishment from the government, or he could commit suicide. There was no third option, at least in his eyes. Therefore, he decided to take his life. But there was hope. Paul screamed from his prison cell, *"Do not harm yourself, for we are all here..."*

In this man's darkest hour, he was given LIGHT. HOPE. A SECOND CHANCE. He was given an opportunity to get to know Jesus. He asked a question that maybe you need to ask. His question was this...

"Sirs, what must I do to be saved?"

He was given the answer, *"Believe in the Lord Jesus, and you will be saved, you and your household."* That belief encompassed him learning the facts about Jesus. It required him to repent of his sins. It required him to be baptized for the forgiveness of sins. This man would receive the saving grace of God and be delivered from his sins!

He was able to lay aside the weight that he truly needed to release. Jesus transformed this man's life. Jesus can transform your life too. Maybe you've been focusing way too much on the scale instead of dealing with your relationship with God. If so, now is the time for you to lay aside the weight. Will you do what this man did? Will you do what Paul did in Acts 22:16 where a man named Ananias told him, *"Now why do you delay? Get up and be baptized, and wash away your sins, calling on his name."*

A relationship with God is how we will go beyond the scale. Instead of focusing so much on letting go of the weight, let's be sure that we also are focused on what we need to be putting on. The apostle Paul reminds us that we need to put on Christ, Galatians 3:26-27.

"For you are all sons of God through faith in Christ Jesus. For all of you who were baptized into Christ have clothed yourselves with Christ."

We put on Christ through baptism. Be sure you really understand what you really look like. You bear the image of God. In Matthew 22:21, Jesus said,

"Render to Caesar the things that are Caesar's and to God the things that are God's." You ultimately belong to God. You bear His image. In the context, the coin presented to Jesus bared the image of Caesar. Just as that piece of money the Jews were to give to Caesar bore his image, Jesus was saying to them, "You bear the image of God. Therefore, give yourselves entirely to Him. Are you ready to do that?

Answer Yes or No. _____

Chapter Fourteen: Exercise Does Profit a Little

"For bodily exercises profits only a little…"

Many Christians are familiar with what Paul said in 1 Timothy 4:8. Here's what he said.

> "…for bodily discipline is only of little profit, but godliness is profitable for all things, since it holds promise for the present life and also for the life to come."

Some sometimes use this verse to get out of exercising. While it can be funny to make light of the fact of what Paul said concerning bodily exercise, there are a few things to consider.

First, Paul was probably in good physical condition. People in the first century were physically active. They didn't really have a choice. They did a lot of walking. One example I often think about with Paul is found in Acts 20. As Paul was headed to Assos, we see that he took a little stroll. Okay, it was more than just a short walk. The text says in Acts 20:13-14

> "But we, going ahead to the ship, set sail for Assos, intending from there to take Paul on board; for so he had arranged it, intending himself to go by land. And when he met us at Assos, we took him on board and came to Mitylene."

Paul probably walked about 20 miles. I don't know if Paul wanted some down time to be alone or to perhaps to pray. I don't know if he intended to talk to people along the way. What I do know is that Paul had to be in good physical condition to walk 20 miles. Why am I saying this?

I'm saying it because exercise does profit…a little. When compared with godliness, it's not on the same level. Yet, as we strive to become more devoted to the Lord, and His work, it's essential that we take care of our bodies. There are many reasons as to why we should be concerned with our health.

- When we maintain a healthy weight, we will have more energy to do God's work.
- It demonstrates self-control and discipline in our lives.

- When you get into shape and take better care of your body, it begins to have a ripple effect in other parts of your life.
- It will help you to save money on healthcare (the name of the game is to stay out of the hospital).
- You will be leaving behind a health and fitness legacy to your children. That's a huge deal. Our children often imitate what they see us doing. Sadly, so many children are already battling with health issues due to being overweight.
- From a husband and wife perspective, it is a way of honoring your spouse. For many of us, when we got married, we were not 10, 20, 30, or 50 pounds overweight. While our marriages are more than about the physical attraction, physical attraction is also significant. Wouldn't you agree?

A little bit of exercise will be able to go a long way. Don't ignore what Paul is saying about godliness. Godliness is what we need to be paying great attention to. Yet bodily exercise does profit a little.

Chapter Fifteen: Where's My Exercise Routine and Eating Plan?

"The muscle you need to first exercise and feed is your mind!"

Okay, now it's time to workout! But we're not going to start with the dumbbells or the treadmill. As I thought about how I wanted to put this book together, I decided that the first muscle we must get into shape is our mindset. I have included in this book space for you to journal. This journal is designed to help you get your mind focused on the right things. Here's what is in that section:

> Motivational thoughts from me to help you along the way.
> Space for you to write out your prayers.
> An area for you to list what you're grateful for in your life.
> Space to will allow you to journal about your day, how you're feeling, successes you've had, challenges, and how you can improve the next day.

As you do this journal, be honest with yourself. If you're struggling with something, write it down. If you've had a great day, write it down. Focus on the positives. Some may think to do this is a little silly, but I don't. It's better than all of the negative stuff we often say to ourselves. I've come to love writing out my thoughts. It helps to clear my mind, and it also helps to see where I may need to pivot and adjust. You can do this in the morning time, afternoon, or evening. Whatever suits you the best. Just be sure to do it. Becoming intentional will give you a gentle push to accomplishing your goals. Before you begin, I want to provide you with a few more suggestions to help you along your journey.

> ***Find a program and stick to it.*** When it comes to going Beyond the Scale, you will need to find a good exercise regimen. I have provided a more extensive list of ideas for you at the end of this book. But for now, one tip I would like to give you is the importance of staying consistent. Here's what I mean. When you start a program, stick to it. Give yourself 4, 8,12, or 52 weeks before you decide to jump ship. Too many times people get started with something and then quickly give up on it. That's silly. You must learn to follow through. If you want personal help, then feel free to reach out to me.
> ***Find a community that will help you along the way.*** When it comes to fitness, there is strength in numbers. There's a great benefit of

being a part of a group of people who will encourage you and motivate you along the way. I'm not saying that you can't work out by yourself or even accomplish a lot of your goals by doing it alone. You certainly can. However, for many people, they often need some kind of assistance. I recommend that you sign up at a local gym, become a part of a cross-fit group, or maybe start a walking club in your neighborhood. The point is, connect with others. There are lots of exercise groups on Facebook (I have one too). The more you can surround yourself with others going in the same direction as you, the stronger you will become. Think about how Christ has designed local churches. There's a plurality of people. They are to encourage one another, <u>Hebrews 10:23-24</u>. The text says, *Let us hold fast the confession of our hope without wavering, for He who promised is faithful; and let us consider how to stimulate one another to love and good deeds...* There is strength in numbers. Christians who don't associate with other Christians are going to fail. Christians who don't see the importance of being a part of a local church will not survive. The same typically happens when it comes to fitness goals. Join a club or start your own.

Know you will be successful. You can do this. I believe in you. But you need to believe in yourself. You can make the necessary changes to get where you want to be. It will take time. It will take effort. It will take persistence. The point is this: It can be done. Therefore, there are NO EXCUSES. Let's go.

Additional Resources

Motivational Journal

Day 1: "You can do it. Get the ball rolling right now ..."

Write out a prayer to the Lord.

What are you thankful for today? How will you demonstrate gratitude today?

How are you feeling? Write out any thoughts, successes, challenges you had today. Be honest with yourself. What can you learn from what you experienced?

Day 2: "Take a before photo to see where you are beginning. Vow to make this the last time you ever take one."

Write out a prayer to the Lord.

What are you thankful for today? How will you demonstrate gratitude today?

How are you feeling? Write out any thoughts, successes, challenges you had today. Be honest with yourself. What can you learn from what you experienced?

Day 3: "No more wasting time. We've already done enough of that. Let's go."

Write out a prayer to the Lord.

What are you thankful for today? How will you demonstrate gratitude today?

How are you feeling? Write out any thoughts, successes, challenges you had today. Be honest with yourself. What can you learn from what you experienced?

Day 4: "This is all up to you. You get to decide the results you will have."

Write out a prayer to the Lord.

What are you thankful for today? How will you demonstrate gratitude today?

How are you feeling? Write out any thoughts, successes, challenges you had today. Be honest with yourself. What can you learn from what you experienced?

Day 5: "This is a journey we're on. Enjoy each day. You can do it."
Write out a prayer to the Lord.

What are you thankful for today? How will you demonstrate gratitude today?

How are you feeling? Write out any thoughts, successes, challenges you had today. Be honest with yourself. What can you learn from what you experienced?

Day 6: "Follow through with your commitment."

Write out a prayer to the Lord.

What are you thankful for today? How will you demonstrate gratitude today?

How are you feeling? Write out any thoughts, successes, challenges you had today. Be honest with yourself. What can you learn from what you experienced?

Day 7: "This is about action. You either want it, or you don't. Let's go."
Write out a prayer to the Lord.

What are you thankful for today? How will you demonstrate gratitude today?

How are you feeling? Write out any thoughts, successes, challenges you had today. Be honest with yourself. What can you learn from what you experienced?

Day 8: "Every workout needs to be done like it's your last. You have to push and do more."

Write out a prayer to the Lord.

What are you thankful for today? How will you demonstrate gratitude today?

How are you feeling? Write out any thoughts, successes, challenges you had today. Be honest with yourself. What can you learn from what you experienced?

Day 9: *"People will try to hold you back. Don't let them. Just keep going."*

Write out a prayer to the Lord.

What are you thankful for today? How will you demonstrate gratitude today?

How are you feeling? Write out any thoughts, successes, challenges you had today. Be honest with yourself. What can you learn from what you experienced?

Day 10: "You are getting closer. Don't stop now."

Write out a prayer to the Lord.

What are you thankful for today? How will you demonstrate gratitude today?

How are you feeling? Write out any thoughts, successes, challenges you had today. Be honest with yourself. What can you learn from what you experienced?

Day 11: *"You have to push yourself like never before. Even when life gets tough."*

Write out a prayer to the Lord.

What are you thankful for today? How will you demonstrate gratitude today?

How are you feeling? Write out any thoughts, successes, challenges you had today. Be honest with yourself. What can you learn from what you experienced?

Day 12: "Talk good to yourself. Quit beating yourself up so much."
Write out a prayer to the Lord.

What are you thankful for today? How will you demonstrate gratitude today?

How are you feeling? Write out any thoughts, successes, challenges you had today. Be honest with yourself. What can you learn from what you experienced?

Day 13: "Do the simple things like preparing and planning your meals, exercising 5–6 days a week, and eating healthy. Results will follow."

Write out a prayer to the Lord.

What are you thankful for today? How will you demonstrate gratitude today?

How are you feeling? Write out any thoughts, successes, challenges you had today. Be honest with yourself. What can you learn from what you experienced?

Day 14: "You get to decide how successful you will be. Don't give up. Keep fighting. C'mon."

Write out a prayer to the Lord.

What are you thankful for today? How will you demonstrate gratitude today?

How are you feeling? Write out any thoughts, successes, challenges you had today. Be honest with yourself. What can you learn from what you experienced?

Day 15: "Allow others to help you along the way. Receive compliments with a smile. You can't do this by yourself."

Write out a prayer to the Lord.

What are you thankful for today? How will you demonstrate gratitude today?

How are you feeling? Write out any thoughts, successes, challenges you had today. Be honest with yourself. What can you learn from what you experienced?

Day 16: "Every day is a step in the right direction." Just keep going."
Write out a prayer to the Lord.

What are you thankful for today? How will you demonstrate gratitude today?

How are you feeling? Write out any thoughts, successes, challenges you had today. Be honest with yourself. What can you learn from what you experienced?

Day 17: "Get out of your own way."

Write out a prayer to the Lord.

What are you thankful for today? How will you demonstrate gratitude today?

How are you feeling? Write out any thoughts, successes, challenges you had today. Be honest with yourself. What can you learn from what you experienced?

Day 18: "Take the time to give yourself a pat on the back with the good work you've been doing."

Write out a prayer to the Lord.

What are you thankful for today? How will you demonstrate gratitude today?

How are you feeling? Write out any thoughts, successes, challenges you had today. Be honest with yourself. What can you learn from what you experienced?

Day 19: "Releasing the weight takes time. Be patient. We are not going after quick fixes."

Write out a prayer to the Lord.

What are you thankful for today? How will you demonstrate gratitude today?

How are you feeling? Write out any thoughts, successes, challenges you had today. Be honest with yourself. What can you learn from what you experienced?

Day 20: "Think about where you want to be one year from now. It will take some time, but you will get there."

Write out a prayer to the Lord.

What are you thankful for today? How will you demonstrate gratitude today?

How are you feeling? Write out any thoughts, successes, challenges you had today. Be honest with yourself. What can you learn from what you experienced?

Day 21: "This is about you changing once and for all."

Write out a prayer to the Lord.

What are you thankful for today? How will you demonstrate gratitude today?

How are you feeling? Write out any thoughts, successes, challenges you had today. Be honest with yourself. What can you learn from what you experienced?

Day 22: "Celebrate your victories. You've put in the hard work. You can do it."

Write out a prayer to the Lord.

What are you thankful for today? How will you demonstrate gratitude today?

How are you feeling? Write out any thoughts, successes, challenges you had today. Be honest with yourself. What can you learn from what you experienced?

Day 23: *"The results will come. Don't stop now. Let's go."*

Write out a prayer to the Lord.

What are you thankful for today? How will you demonstrate gratitude today?

How are you feeling? Write out any thoughts, successes, challenges you had today. Be honest with yourself. What can you learn from what you experienced?

Day 24: "Expect the best, and you will often get it."

Write out a prayer to the Lord.

What are you thankful for today? How will you demonstrate gratitude today?

How are you feeling? Write out any thoughts, successes, challenges you had today. Be honest with yourself. What can you learn from what you experienced?

Day 25: "A positive mindset is key. Fill your mind with good thoughts. Get rid of the junk."

Write out a prayer to the Lord.

What are you thankful for today? How will you demonstrate gratitude today?

How are you feeling? Write out any thoughts, successes, challenges you had today. Be honest with yourself. What can you learn from what you experienced?

Day 26: *"You have to stay hungry. You have to want it. Let's go, baby.*

Write out a prayer to the Lord.

What are you thankful for today? How will you demonstrate gratitude today?

How are you feeling? Write out any thoughts, successes, challenges you had today. Be honest with yourself. What can you learn from what you experienced?

110

Day 27: "If you keep going, you will thank yourself three, six, nine, and 12 months from now. Just keep going.

Write out a prayer to the Lord.

What are you thankful for today? How will you demonstrate gratitude today?

How are you feeling? Write out any thoughts, successes, challenges you had today. Be honest with yourself. What can you learn from what you experienced?

Day 28: "Someone is counting on you. You can do it. Focus!
Write out a prayer to the Lord.

What are you thankful for today? How will you demonstrate gratitude today?

How are you feeling? Write out any thoughts, successes, challenges you had today. Be honest with yourself. What can you learn from what you experienced?

112

Day 29: "There can be NO EXCUSES. We're all busy. Find a way."

Write out a prayer to the Lord.

What are you thankful for today? How will you demonstrate gratitude today?

How are you feeling? Write out any thoughts, successes, challenges you had today. Be honest with yourself. What can you learn from what you experienced?

Day 30: "Great job staying strong for 30 days. Now do it again. And again."

Write out a prayer to the Lord.

What are you thankful for today? How will you demonstrate gratitude today?

How are you feeling? Write out any thoughts, successes, challenges you had today. Be honest with yourself. What can you learn from what you experienced?

Day 31: There's someone right now who would love to be in your shoes! There is someone who would like to be able to put on those workout clothes, sit in traffic, endure the cold weather, and wake up early to go to the gym to workout.

They would love to feel sweaty. They would love to stand upright and flex in the mirror. They would like to experience the feeling of running, of doing push-ups, or gripping weights.

Don't take for granted what you can do. Many would love to have weights in their house! Take nothing for granted! Get up, go, work, sweat, rejoice and no complaining! Take nothing for granted!

Write out a prayer to the Lord.

What are you thankful for today? How will you demonstrate gratitude today?

How are you feeling? Write out any thoughts, successes, challenges you had today. Be honest with yourself. What can you learn from what you experienced?

Day 32: Embrace the challenge! Whether it's the holiday season or the middle of June, you need to do the impossible or at least the impossible in the eyes of many. You need to stay on track. Who cares if it is the holiday season. Who cares if you are on vacation. Who cares if you are busy. You must find a way.

Life is a challenge, so go ahead and embrace it. Eating healthy while traveling is a challenge. Eating healthy while taking care of children is a challenge. Embrace the challenge. Eating healthy and working out even when you don't want to is a challenge. Embrace the challenge and crush it.

You are going to eat clean. You are going to lose weight and build muscle. You are going to change your body for life. This must become an obsession. Think about it, breathe it, live it, crush it.

Write out a prayer to the Lord.

What are you thankful for today? How will you demonstrate gratitude today?

How are you feeling? Write out any thoughts, successes, challenges you had today. Be honest with yourself. What can you learn from what you experienced?

Day 33: It's time for work! It's time for a change! It's time for strength! It's time to flourish! It's time for explosive change! It's time, baby! It's time, baby! It's time to break through!

Write out a prayer to the Lord.

What are you thankful for today? How will you demonstrate gratitude today?

How are you feeling? Write out any thoughts, successes, challenges you had today. Be honest with yourself. What can you learn from what you experienced?

Day 34: Transformation is about change. You can't remain the same. You must push forward, and leave the past in the past. Remember, every day is another opportunity for you to change. But you must decide you are ready to pay the price it will take to improve. The sacrifice will be worth it.

Write out a prayer to the Lord.

What are you thankful for today? How will you demonstrate gratitude today?

How are you feeling? Write out any thoughts, successes, challenges you had today. Be honest with yourself. What can you learn from what you experienced?

Day 35: Keep it going. Don't give up. Get up and go exercise. Motivate yourself, and remember your goals.

Write out a prayer to the Lord.

What are you thankful for today? How will you demonstrate gratitude today?

How are you feeling? Write out any thoughts, successes, challenges you had today. Be honest with yourself. What can you learn from what you experienced?

Day 36: Get out of your own way, and be victorious. Allow yourself to be successful. Don't be afraid to accomplish your goals. Go get them!!! Right now!

It's time to crank it out like never before. There can be no excuses. It doesn't matter if you have to travel a lot. That's not an excuse for you to sabotage your efforts. Failure is not an option. There are people who need you to be strong.

Every day you decide to make a change, you will become stronger. Don't be afraid of success. Don't sabotage all of your hard work. Keep going.

Write out a prayer to the Lord.

What are you thankful for today? How will you demonstrate gratitude today?

How are you feeling? Write out any thoughts, successes, challenges you had today. Be honest with yourself. What can you learn from what you experienced?

Day 37: Don't wait for anybody...Just Go!

Write out a prayer to the Lord.

What are you thankful for today? How will you demonstrate gratitude today?

How are you feeling? Write out any thoughts, successes, challenges you had today. Be honest with yourself. What can you learn from what you experienced?

Day 38: If you want to get something, you will have to pay the fee. You will have to say "No" to get to your "Yes."

Write out a prayer to the Lord.

What are you thankful for today? How will you demonstrate gratitude today?

How are you feeling? Write out any thoughts, successes, challenges you had today. Be honest with yourself. What can you learn from what you experienced?

Day 39: I found some more leverage in my closet! A suit I haven't worn in a really long time! I was thinking, "I wonder if it fits?" It does! Clothes don't lie. Neither does the mirror.

Find what you need to stay focused! Is it that holiday party? That dress? That suit? Is it your children? What can you find today that will help you to stay on track? Whatever it is, use it.

Write out a prayer to the Lord.

What are you thankful for today? How will you demonstrate gratitude today?

How are you feeling? Write out any thoughts, successes, challenges you had today. Be honest with yourself. What can you learn from what you experienced?

Day 40: No more before photos. Push it. Do more. Make sure you don't go back. Don't go back to being lazy, wishing but never taking action. Don't quit. Remember what you told yourself you would do on Day 1. Be sure to keep the commitment you made.

Write out a prayer to the Lord.

What are you thankful for today? How will you demonstrate gratitude today?

How are you feeling? Write out any thoughts, successes, challenges you had today. Be honest with yourself. What can you learn from what you experienced?

Day 41: It's time to take it up another notch! You only can control what you can control! But you can control a lot.

Write out a prayer to the Lord.

What are you thankful for today? How will you demonstrate gratitude today?

How are you feeling? Write out any thoughts, successes, challenges you had today. Be honest with yourself. What can you learn from what you experienced?

Day 42: Transforming and making real changes requires you to keep a positive mindset. During this process, you will have to talk to yourself positively. That's part of motivating yourself.

Write out a prayer to the Lord.

What are you thankful for today? How will you demonstrate gratitude today?

How are you feeling? Write out any thoughts, successes, challenges you had today. Be honest with yourself. What can you learn from what you experienced?

Day 43: There will be times when life will be challenging. Life happens! But somehow you are going to have to find a way. This may require you to wake up earlier than usual. Or you may need to stay up later than usual, so you can get in that workout. When life gets busy, you might get a little too relaxed with exercise and your time with God. You can't allow that to happen. Find a way.

Write out a prayer to the Lord.

What are you thankful for today? How will you demonstrate gratitude today?

How are you feeling? Write out any thoughts, successes, challenges you had today. Be honest with yourself. What can you learn from what you experienced?

Day 44: Let's face, you know how to eat! Sometimes you can eat like there will not be a tomorrow. But breathe, and take a step back from that cookie or cinnamon roll. Do you really need to eat that? Don't worry, you can say "NO" now, so you can say "YES" later. The food is not going anywhere. Stay on track.

Write out a prayer to the Lord.

What are you thankful for today? How will you demonstrate gratitude today?

How are you feeling? Write out any thoughts, successes, challenges you had today. Be honest with yourself. What can you learn from what you experienced?

Day 45: This journey to better health and a better life is not merely about you. People are watching you right now. Yes, that's right. Don't let them down.

Write out a prayer to the Lord.

What are you thankful for today? How will you demonstrate gratitude today?

How are you feeling? Write out any thoughts, successes, challenges you had today. Be honest with yourself. What can you learn from what you experienced?

Day 46: I will honor my promises. I will transform for LIFE. I will keep my commitments to God. I will keep my obligations to my family. I WILL...Go ahead and say it with me... "I WILL SUCCEED."

Write out a prayer to the Lord.

What are you thankful for today? How will you demonstrate gratitude today?

How are you feeling? Write out any thoughts, successes, challenges you had today. Be honest with yourself. What can you learn from what you experienced?

Day 47: Do as much as you can. Have no regrets.

Write out a prayer to the Lord.

What are you thankful for today? How will you demonstrate gratitude today?

How are you feeling? Write out any thoughts, successes, challenges you had today. Be honest with yourself. What can you learn from what you experienced?

Day 48: Do you realize how blessed you really are? Has the gratitude list been helping you? Indeed, you are blessed. The fact that you have life and the ability to exercise is a reason for you to be thankful. Don't take for granted the opportunities you have right in front of you.

Write out a prayer to the Lord.

What are you thankful for today? How will you demonstrate gratitude today?

How are you feeling? Write out any thoughts, successes, challenges you had today. Be honest with yourself. What can you learn from what you experienced?

Day 49: Don't fumble the ball at the one-yard line. Go all the way into the end zone. Finish what you have started.

Write out a prayer to the Lord.

What are you thankful for today? How will you demonstrate gratitude today?

How are you feeling? Write out any thoughts, successes, challenges you had today. Be honest with yourself. What can you learn from what you experienced?

Day 50: You are in the no excuse zone. All excuses have to be put to the side. Besides, no one really wants to hear excuses.

Write out a prayer to the Lord.

What are you thankful for today? How will you demonstrate gratitude today?

How are you feeling? Write out any thoughts, successes, challenges you had today. Be honest with yourself. What can you learn from what you experienced?

Day 51: It's easy to zoom in on everything that is wrong. But that will accomplish very little. Focus on what is right. Then you will be alright.

Write out a prayer to the Lord.

What are you thankful for today? How will you demonstrate gratitude today?

How are you feeling? Write out any thoughts, successes, challenges you had today. Be honest with yourself. What can you learn from what you experienced?

Day 52: Everyone has an "It." It is that moment when life punches you in the face. You are not the exception. We all go through something. Therefore, we must keep going.

Write out a prayer to the Lord.

What are you thankful for today? How will you demonstrate gratitude today?

How are you feeling? Write out any thoughts, successes, challenges you had today. Be honest with yourself. What can you learn from what you experienced?

136

Day 53: There can be no quit. Get better today.

Write out a prayer to the Lord.

What are you thankful for today? How will you demonstrate gratitude today?

How are you feeling? Write out any thoughts, successes, challenges you had today. Be honest with yourself. What can you learn from what you experienced?

Day 54: What if you worked out as much as you watched television? Turn the television off and go exercise.

Write out a prayer to the Lord.

What are you thankful for today? How will you demonstrate gratitude today?

How are you feeling? Write out any thoughts, successes, challenges you had today. Be honest with yourself. What can you learn from what you experienced?

Day 55: No more quick fixes and weird diets. Just work hard.

Write out a prayer to the Lord.

What are you thankful for today? How will you demonstrate gratitude today?

How are you feeling? Write out any thoughts, successes, challenges you had today. Be honest with yourself. What can you learn from what you experienced?

Day 56: It's a new day! Make the most of it.

Write out a prayer to the Lord.

What are you thankful for today? How will you demonstrate gratitude today?

How are you feeling? Write out any thoughts, successes, challenges you had today. Be honest with yourself. What can you learn from what you experienced?

Day 57: Tired of losing the same weight over and over? Not doing it anymore. How much weight have you lost? 100 pounds? Some would say, "no way." But if you're losing the same 20 pounds every two years over a decade that's 100 pounds. C'mon! Are you fed up yet? Change your language. Instead of "losing weight" how about releasing the weight once and for all.

Write out a prayer to the Lord.

What are you thankful for today? How will you demonstrate gratitude today?

How are you feeling? Write out any thoughts, successes, challenges you had today. Be honest with yourself. What can you learn from what you experienced?

Day 58: The waistline won't shrink on its own. The muscles won't develop overnight. You must put in the work. So go do it now!

Write out a prayer to the Lord.

What are you thankful for today? How will you demonstrate gratitude today?

How are you feeling? Write out any thoughts, successes, challenges you had today. Be honest with yourself. What can you learn from what you experienced?

Day 59: When adversity hits you in the gut...When stressful times come rolling in like a thunderstorm...When disappointment moves into your house and doesn't seem to leave...Be sure you turn to God.

Write out a prayer to the Lord.

What are you thankful for today? How will you demonstrate gratitude today?

How are you feeling? Write out any thoughts, successes, challenges you had today. Be honest with yourself. What can you learn from what you experienced?

Day 60: Rain or shine. Sleep or no sleep. Stressed or relaxed. Busy or bored. Hungry or full. Crying or laughing. Day or night. Employed or unemployed. Get your workout in .If you can walk, then walk, if you can run then run, if you can lift them lift. C'mon now. Yeah, I'm talking to you! There's no turning back!

Write out a prayer to the Lord.

What are you thankful for today? How will you demonstrate gratitude today?

How are you feeling? Write out any thoughts, successes, challenges you had today. Be honest with yourself. What can you learn from what you experienced?

I Just Wrote Your Eulogy.

_____ was ____ years old when (he/she) passed from this side of life.

_____is survived by (his/her) spouse _____and their children _____.

The Bible says that it is appointed for men to die once and after that the judgment in <u>Hebrews 9:27</u>.

Life is a journey that will eventually end. Death is also a journey that will lead our souls into eternity.

_____ is now in the realm of the unseen. (His/her) fate is sealed.

_____will stand before a just God.

The God of Abraham, Isaac, and Jacob is described as the righteous judge in <u>Genesis 18:25</u>.

God is also described as the God of all comfort, the faithful Creator, and the one who can't lie. _____ is in good hands.

Death is not the end, but merely the beginning. While that's true, it's never easy for family to lose a loved one.

I know how you all cared for _____.

I pray for the family at this time that God will comfort you in your time of sorrow. Take your time with grieving. The Israelites mourned for 30 days after Moses died, <u>Deuteronomy 34:8</u>.

Everyone's grief is unique, <u>Proverbs 14:10</u>. There will be people who will say, "I know how you feel…" but they don't. But God does! Praise God for that.

Cling to Him when your eyes are filled with tears. Turn to Him when you become weak, and don't know how you will move forward.

In America, we rush too much with death and mourning. We're back to work after taking a few days off (if we have vacation time). Our schedules are too busy. To the family, allow yourself time to cry, vent, and do nothing! But there is something else to consider…

While Israel mourned for Moses, they still had to do something. Eventually, they had to keep pressing forward. There were still blessings ahead for them to possess. You too in your own time must do the same. You will have to continue living. It doesn't mean you have to stop grieving, but it does mean you have to keep living.

The sun will continue to rise and to set. Holidays will come and go. Seasons will continue to come and go. You must continue.

But this doesn't mean that you should move on from the memories, experiences, and joy you had with _____. Hold on to those memories.

_____ was a person of faith. It was clear who _____ served…God.

_____ was in love with (his/her) family, and they loved (him/her) very much.

_____ had (his/her) priorities in order…

Faith…

Family…

Then everything else!

_____ was sacrificial with (his/her) time. There were times when _____ turned down overtime at work so (he/she) could really LIVE LIFE.

Speaking of living life, it appeared that _____ really did enjoy life!

Concerning life, one person said, "Many are alive, but many are not truly living!" That was not the case for _____.

_____ was in great shape. However, _____ recognized that there's more to life than just exercising every day. But (he/she) also realized that (his/her) health was important as (he/she) strived to give honor to God in all things and to be there for (his/her) family.

_____ strived to leave a spiritual legacy for (his/her) family.

(He/she) practiced what (he/she) taught others. It was clear _____ was seeking first the kingdom of God, Matthew 6:33.

Now _____ made mistakes like everyone else. But it was clear that ____ had a heart of repentance, and learned from their mistakes.

_____ children really loved (him/her). They were always excited seeing (him/her).

_____ spouse loved (him/her) so much. It was clear that _____ gave (his/her) spouse the honor they deserved and that God expected.

_____ was giving of (his/her) time with volunteering and assisting others. People in the community saw (him/her) treating (his/her) neighbors the right way.

_____ light shined! People wanted to know what gave _____ great joy and peace. (His/her) answer was, "I know who I am in Christ."

_____ was in Christ. _____ put Christ on as Paul instructed in Galatians 3:27.

_____ knew about the power of the gospel, and obeyed it to receive God's grace, Romans 1:16, 10:17, 3:23, 10:9-10, 6:1-4, 7, 23.

_____ did what Jesus said to do in Mark 16:16.

I do know that, and I take great comfort in knowing that. To the family, take comfort in that also.

_____ was able to love life and see good days. _____ family has followed in (his/her) footsteps seeking to honor God with their lives.

May God Bless the family! _____ loved you, and God loves you too.

End of your Eulogy.

So, what do you think? To much? Over the top? Not enough said?

Did you put your name in the blanks? Good! Now ask yourself this question...

"Could a preacher say those things about you at your funeral?" If not, why not? I have to ask and answer the same question myself. Have you thought what might be said at your funeral? Every day you get to decide what can be said. Everyday WE get to choose, by our attitudes, actions, and aspirations in our lives. Many don't think about their funeral. Many don't think about the cost and preparation that goes into a funeral for the family.

We should. Jacob gave instructions to his family, with what to do with his body after he died, <u>Genesis 50:1-6</u>.

In the end, when we're dead, we will not hear what someone will say about us.

Let's be more concerned with how we're living now, treating others, and living for God.

Let's be concerned with what God will say to us on Judgment Day!

I can't write your Eulogy…

But YOU CAN!!! Make every day count.

Where to Begin in Your Physical Transformation?

I don't know about you, but it can be very intimidating what to listen to and where to begin when it comes to losing weight. If you listen to talk shows, you will see and hear a variety of experts who will tell you what to do. When you walk into a bookstore, you will see numerous exercise and weight loss books. If you listen to the radio, you will hear commercials about the latest diet.

It feels like information overload. I would encourage you to consult with your physician before you begin any kind of program. There can be a variety of factors when it comes to why some people may lose weight faster than others. I make no claims that if these things are done, you will lose what you desire.

Having been a health journey for the last two years, I have observed some things in myself and in others. I want to share those with you. Below is a list of thoughts that may be able to help you as you begin or continue your weight loss journey. You may wish to dive into these a little bit more, or you may want to ignore them. The choice is yours. I wish you the best of luck. God Bless.

What I have learned...

> *Mindset really is key*. A person can have hundreds of books, but until they change their mind, they will have difficulty really making a change.
>
> *Flood your mind with positive thoughts*. I did this with journaling in the morning. I would write out my prayers. I would write out positive thoughts to myself. It doesn't matter if you think they are silly. No one else saw them except me. It worked for me. It may work for you.
>
> *You must be willing to struggle*. When my son was learning how to tie his shoes, he screamed while crying, "I'm struggling so much." He did struggle. But he came out victorious. In your weight loss journey, you will struggle. But if you continue, you will be victorious. Be willing to struggle. Things will not always go as you would like them to. There will be setbacks. That's normal and expected. Quit assuming that things will be perfect. They won't be. Struggle for what it is that you want.

Drink lots of water. As I went through my physical transformation, I was drinking at least 100 ounces of water a day. I'm not going to tell you an exact amount of what you need to drink. But I know this. You need to drink water. It's free. It's what your body needs. Drink up. Replace your sodas with more water. Learn to like the taste of it. Some say drink it warm while others say drink it cold. You decide. Just drink it. Add some lemon juice to it if you like. That's what I began doing. Every morning, I would cut up a lemon and squeeze the juice into my water.

Wake up at the same time. During my transformation, I began focusing a lot more on my sleep. Sleep is important. I think we can get accustomed to being sleep deprived. Get your sleep on. I would also encourage that you wake up at the same time each morning. This may be challenging at times, but eventually, it will become normal. Try to do it also on the weekends. It will require discipline. Discipline is important. Remember, you will have to struggle.

Find a program and stick to it. There are so many fitness books out there. It gets tiring trying to find out which one to follow. My recommendation is to find one that fits where you are and something that will be sustainable. Try something for at least a couple of months. See if it will work for you. But be careful that you don't fall into the "I want to lose weight instantly trap." So many fall into this category, and as a result, they will do something extreme. They will see some achievements along the way, but in the process of time, their bodies will rebound. This can and may begin a terrible cycle of weight loss and weight gain. Back and forth. No fun. Waste of time. Avoid this. If you want simple things you can do if you don't want to look at specific programs, here you go.

> *Move every day:* As humans, we are designed to move. Yet so many people live sedentary lives. You need to move. Take a walk every day. That's free. If you can't walk, then get on a bike or find a place to go swimming. This is basic and free. If you can jog or run, begin going for a jog on a daily basis. Start slow and build your endurance. This could be where you run to the end of the street and then back home. The next day go a little further and continue to build from that. You will be amazed at how quickly your endurance will grow. Your cardio sessions do not have to be long. Try to go for 10 or 15 minutes. This will serve

you well. For the last few years, I've done High-Intensity Interval Training. I will do this outside or on my spin bike. I will walk for two minutes. Then I will jog for two minutes. Then I will run as fast as I can for one minute. Then I start the process all over again. Do this for 20-30 minutes, and you will be good to go. Maybe you can't go that long. That's okay. Start slow and continue to build. Jump rope and performing burpees are also killer workouts. Again, these kinds of exercises are simple to do and can be done in the home. I typically will do cardio two to three days a week. You don't have to do it every day. Even if you did one day a week, it would be better than nothing. But you have to take that first step and get moving. If you have specific physical challenges then maybe some like Yoga or Pilates might be better for you. You can buy a cheap video on Amazon and perform these exercises in your home. There really are no excuses.

Begin Resistance Training: Start lifting weights. If you're a woman, don't believe the lie that you will get super big. Resistance training is good for both men and women. If you don't have any weights that's okay. Start off by doing some basic push-ups. If you can't do regular push-ups, there are plenty of modifications for you to do. Push-ups are free. You can beat that. You can do air squats to help strengthen your legs. You can do a variety of planks to help improve your core. All of these movements are free and can be looked up online. I love having my own gym in my garage. If I can't make it to the health club, I can simply walk into my garage and get a great workout in. Boom. Simple. Powerful. Effective. Go to Amazon and buy a flat bench or an incline bench. Go to somewhere like Wal-Mart or Academy to purchase some dumbbells. That's all you really need to start your home gym. It's always important that as you train with weights, that you have proper form. If you've never worked out, then be sure to hire a personal trainer or workout with a friend that will be able to guide you in the right direction.

Track your eating and exercise. Keeping track of what you're doing is also really important. Sometimes people are just lazy. They complain about keeping a journal. Then when things aren't working out, they are not able to go back and review what they did or did not do. Don't waste time. Track what you're doing. Your future self will thank you. Go buy a simple journal at the store to track what you're doing. If you want something better than that, then purchase my Faith, Family, Fitness, Food 31 Day Motivational Journal. Buy about three of these. This will help you get on your way. If you need a reminder to eat your meals on a regular basis, use your phone as an alarm to remind you.

Be a part of a team. Look to be a part of some kind of team. Maybe it's a workout group on Facebook. Create your own Facebook group. There is always room for more because everyone has a story to tell. Everyone has a way of helping others. Or join a running group in your town. Whatever it may be, align yourself with some kind of team. You will need the encouragement along the way. Be a part of a team.

Get out of your own way. Sometimes we are our worst enemy. We tell ourselves lies. We convince ourselves with the "If only..." lie. If we only had more time. If we had more knowledge. If we had more people to push us. We all have the same amount of time. We all have plenty of experience. You know there is some benefit of moving your body. That's how they are designed. They are designed to move and not be sedentary all day. You will not always have someone screaming at you to run. You will have to develop an inner drive. This may take some time, but if you follow through with the things I mentioned earlier, it will happen.

Take time off. It's interesting that so many people don't use all of their vacation time on a yearly basis. When I was in pharmaceutical sales, I would always take my vacation time. But for many, they feel the need to work continually. Learn to take some time off. Relax. Take a day off from exercising as well. You will be okay. Mix up your eating from time to time. Enjoy some cake and ice cream on your birthday. You will be fine. Going through my transformation, I would enjoy a few meals each week where I would eat anything. Call them whatever you want to call them. Sometimes I would have a free day. I would purposely eat as much as I wanted to. It was great. It still is. It helps you mentally and probably physically. Take some time off from your regular eating habits. Enjoy some different things. You will be okay.

Buy new clothes when you lose weight. There's something so great about buying new clothes when you lose weight. It helps you to see that progress is being made. Do it. Save some money and get some new clothes.

Throw away your old clothes. After you buy some new clothes, be sure that you throw away those old clothes. Yep, that's right. Get rid of those old clothes. That's what I did. I laid them out. I recognized just how far I had come. I then took them to goodwill or gave them to a friend. It was a great feeling. Leaving them in your closet to me is dangerous. You may be tempted to start wearing them again after you've overeaten knowing that they will be really loose. Don't do that.

Take photos every day. I take a lot of selfies. There are a lot of running jokes from my friends and from people at church because of all the photos that I take. That's okay. Pictures are powerful. I take them as a way of accountability. It's a way to show others that I have worked out. It's a way for me to see what I've done. It's a way to look at your progress or your regression. After a year of photos, you will have a good record of what it is that you have done. Take pictures in the bathroom if you are too shy to take them in the gym area. Just take them. You can keep your clothes on as well.

Find different ways to motivate yourself. I have done some weird things (at least in the eyes of others) to drive myself. But you have to do what you have to do. Below are some of the things I have done to keep myself motivated.

> ***Make your own clothing challenge***. I created the brown suit challenge for myself. Remember the suit I mentioned to you earlier that I couldn't get into? Eventually, I got back into it. One Sunday evening at church during a sermon the preacher told the audience, "Ben has been wearing his brown suit a lot lately. Let's see if he will be able to wear it after Thanksgiving." Challenge accepted! I told the congregation that I would wear the brown suit every Wednesday and Sunday until the end of the year. This was in November of 2016. That's what I did. Maybe you need to create your own challenge. Wear the same clothes to remind yourself that you need to stay in them. It worked for me. Perhaps it will work for you.

Make your own dinner placemat for dinner. Yes, I have done this. I used Shutterfly and made myself a dinner placemat. Here was my thought. If I could see a photo of myself while eating maybe that would help me to maintain my portion control. I know, I know, sounds a little out there. But I had to give it a shot. Maybe it will work for you.

Book a photo shoot. Yes. Do this! It's super powerful to know that you have a deadline. As I mentioned earlier, photos don't lie. This worked well for me. Something else I did with this was marked on my calendar all of the special events I had coming up for the year (holidays, birthdays, anniversaries). I knew I would be taking a lot of photos and I wanted to look my best. This will help you as well.

Make a transformational video. I began doing this using the Splice App. It's fun. Those selfies really started to come in handy. Plus, you never know how this will be able to motivate someone else. Go ahead and give it a shot.

Create your own 5k. A few years ago I got tired of paying a lot of money running in the annual Thanksgiving 5k in my hometown. So I decided to create my own 5k. It was called, "The first annual free 5k Turkey Run." I got first place. However, there were only four runners. But it was fun. I had a friend bring old 5k T-shirts for us to give out. I measured out the distance on my Garmin watch. This first race led to more races and more people. We had one where we had almost 30 people and gift cards donated to us to give out to the winners. Create your own 5k. It's a great way to motivate yourself and others.

One Final Thought

Life is short. Be sure to enjoy it. It's hard to do the things we really want to do when we don't have our health. I'm thankful that you have taken the time to read this book. This has been a labor of love. I never thought that I would write a book like this, but I'm glad I have. If this book helps and motivates one person to draw closer to God, to get into better health, then I will be happy. I would love to hear about your success. Feel free to share with me your great success in life. Now I want you to go forth and be strong. Be courageous. Keep going. Never give up. You have to believe in yourself. I believe in you. You must keep climbing that mountain. You will be successful. God bless you! Stay in touch. If you have any comments or questions, reach out to me at www.benjaminleeonline.com.

51603964R00085

Made in the USA
Columbia, SC
20 February 2019